Studies in Computational Intelligence

Volume 587

Series editor

Janusz Kacprzyk, Polish Academy of Sciences, Warsaw, Poland
e-mail: kacprzyk@ibspan.waw.pl

About this Series

The series "Studies in Computational Intelligence" (SCI) publishes new developments and advances in the various areas of computational intelligence—quickly and with a high quality. The intent is to cover the theory, applications, and design methods of computational intelligence, as embedded in the fields of engineering, computer science, physics and life sciences, as well as the methodologies behind them. The series contains monographs, lecture notes and edited volumes in computational intelligence spanning the areas of neural networks, connectionist systems, genetic algorithms, evolutionary computation, artificial intelligence, cellular automata, self-organizing systems, soft computing, fuzzy systems, and hybrid intelligent systems. Of particular value to both the contributors and the readership are the short publication timeframe and the world-wide distribution, which enable both wide and rapid dissemination of research output.

More information about this series at http://www.springer.com/series/7092

Allan K.Y. Wong · Jackei H.K. Wong
Wilfred W.K. Lin · Tharam S. Dillon
Elizabeth J. Chang

Semantically Based
Clinical TCM
Telemedicine Systems

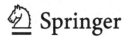 Springer

Allan K.Y. Wong
Department of Computing
Hong Kong Polytechnic University
Hung Hom, Kowloon
Hong Kong SAR

Jackei H.K. Wong
HerbMiners Informatics Limited
Tai Po
Hong Kong SAR

and

Department of Computing
Hong Kong Polytechnic University
Hung Hom, Kowloon
Hong Kong SAR

Wilfred W.K. Lin
HerbMiners Informatics Limited
Tai Po
Hong Kong SAR

and

Department of Computing
Hong Kong Polytechnic University
Hung Hom, Kowloon
Hong Kong SAR

Tharam S. Dillon
Department of Computer Science
  and Computer Engineering
La Trobe University
Melbourne
Australia

Elizabeth J. Chang
School of Business, Australian Defence
  Force Academy
University of New South Wales
Canberra
Australia

ISSN 1860-949X   ISSN 1860-9503   (electronic)
Studies in Computational Intelligence
ISBN 978-3-662-51965-3   ISBN 978-3-662-46024-5   (eBook)
DOI 10.1007/978-3-662-46024-5

Springer Heidelberg New York Dordrecht London

Printed on acid-free paper

Springer-Verlag GmbH Berlin Heidelberg is part of Springer Science+Business Media (www.springer.com)

I dedicate this work to my wife Patricia Hutton, to my world-class colleagues and to all who pursue knowledge.

Allan K.Y. Wong

I dedicate this work to my wife Kathryn Yan, and to the memory of Dr. Allan K.Y. Wong with thanks and admiration.

Jackei H.K. Wong

I dedicate this work to my family and Dr. Allan K.Y. Wong, for his endless support.

Wilfred W.K. Lin

I dedicate this work to my parents Gurdial Singh and Kartar Kaur and to Allan Wong for his vision in initiating this work and his constant friendship.

Tharam S. Dillon

I dedicate this work to my mother Y.Z. Chang and Allan Wong.

Elizabeth J. Chang

Preface

Recent years have seen the development of two significant trends, namely: the adoption of some Traditional Chinese Medicine Practices into mainstream Allopathic Western Medicine; and the advent of the Internet and broadband networks leading to an increased interest in the use of Telemedicine to deliver medical services.

In this book, we see the convergence of these two trends leading to a semantically based TCM Telemedicine system that utilizes an ontology to provide sharable knowledge in the TCM realm to achieve this.

The underpinning research required the development of a three-layer architecture and an Ontology of the TCM knowledge.

As TCM knowledge like all medical knowledge is not frozen in time it was important to develop an approach that would allow evolution of the Ontology when new evidence became available.

In order for the system to be practically grounded it was important to work with an industry partner PuraPharm Group/HerbMiners Informatics Limited. This partnership was initiated through Prof. Allan Wong and the Chairman of PuraPharm Group Mr. Abraham Chan. This led to the system being utilized in more than 20 Mobile Clinics in Hong Kong and 300 Hospitals in China.

In order for these different deployments of the system to be coherent with the main Onto-core it was necessary for us to develop an Ontology-Driven Software System Generation approach.

The organization of the book reflects these issues. We briefly discuss the organization of the book to assist the reader.

Thus Chap. 1 sets out the motivation and significance of the work described in the book. It identifies the main research issues and then provides an overview of the solutions developed in the book.

Chapter 2 gives an explanation of the background knowledge of Traditional Chinese Medicine (TCM) necessary to understand the work of this book, including the evolution of TCM over 3,000 years. It outlines the theoretical framework underlying TCM. It also gives an overview of the diagnostic and treatment approaches employed in TCM. An important issue it highlights is the adoption of TCM treatments in Western Allopathic medicine and the adoption of some western approaches to diagnosis to supplement TCM approaches. It emphasizes the need for a compendium of sharable knowledge in TCM.

Chapter 3 explores the use of the ontology paradigm to capture the semantics and its use as a mechanism for representing Sharable knowledge across a broad community. It also explores techniques for acquiring and conceptual representation of this knowledge. It next examines different approaches to realization of these ontologies in a machine understandable form.

Chapter 4 explores the issues for developing a sharable representation of the TCM knowledge and develops the architecture of the proposed approach.

We utilize an ontology for doing this. Ontologies in general are discussed in Chap. 3. Their use for representing TCM knowledge is discussed in Chap. 4. Thus a TCM Ontology is developed in Chap. 4.

This three-layer architecture for TCM and cross-layer logical transitivity are explained fully in Chap. 4.

We give an overview of this Automatic System Generation Approach in Sect. 1.5 and give a full exposition of it in Chap. 5.

As is the case in Western Allopathic Medicine, in Traditional Chinese Medicine knowledge is constantly being generated as a result of new insights arising from research, clinical practice, experience and observation by TCM practitioners. In order to cater for this growing and evolving knowledge in the field we need mechanisms for evolving the consensus certified knowledge, represented in the TCM Ontology, in a semi-automatic fashion. In Chap. 6, we discuss the framework for such ontology evolution for the TCM Ontology using Mining and a systematic process for updating the Ontology.

In Chap. 7, we describe a model of the Network Infrastructure for delivery of the TCM over the Telemedicine System over the Internet. We carry out a performance analysis of the Telemedicine System based on this model.

Lastly, in Chap. 8, we provide a recapitulation of the work described in this book, summarizing what has been achieved. This is followed by a discussion of the future directions that this research on semantically based TCM Telemedicine can take.

Allan K.Y. Wong
Department of Computing
Hong Kong Polytechnic University

Jackei H.K. Wong
HerbMiners Informatics Limited
Department of Computing
Hong Kong Polytechnic University

Wilfred W.K. Lin
HerbMiners Informatics Limited
Department of Computing
Hong Kong Polytechnic University

Tharam S. Dillon
Department of Computer Science
and Computer Engineering
La Trobe University

Elizabeth J. Chang
School of Business, Australian Defence
Force Academy
University of New South Wales

Contents

1 **Telemedicine and Knowledge Representation for Traditional Chinese Medicine** 1
  1.1 Traditional Chinese Medicine and a Consensus Certified Knowledge Base 1
  1.2 Traditional Chinese Medicine and Telemedicine 2
    1.2.1 What is Telemedicine? 2
    1.2.2 Knowledge Consultation 4
    1.2.3 Curative Aspects 4
    1.2.4 Training by E-Learning 4
    1.2.5 Management and Control 5
    1.2.6 Efficient and Reliable Information Communication Technology (ICT) Support 5
    1.2.7 Explicit Semantics 5
  1.3 Automatic System Generation and Evolution of the TCM Knowledge 7
  1.4 Major Aspects of the Ontology Base TCM Telemedicine System 7
    1.4.1 Ontology Modelling 8
    1.4.2 Ontology Implementation Tool 8
    1.4.3 Internet Capability 9
    1.4.4 Architecture and Cross-layer Logical Transitivity 9
    1.4.5 Automatic System Generation 10
    1.4.6 Pervasive Support 10
    1.4.7 Ontology Evolution Approach 11
  1.5 Overview of the Ontology-Based Automatic System Generation (ASG/C) 12
  1.6 Recapitulation 16
  References 16

2   The TCM Ambit.....................................   19
    2.1   The Evolution of Traditional Chinese Medicine   19
    2.2   Underlying Theory   20
    2.3   TCM Diagnosis and Treatment.........................   22
    2.4   Herbal Pharmacology   24
    2.5   Computer-Aided TCM Takes Various Forms   25
    2.6   Contemporary TCM Telemedicine   27
    References...   28

3   Semantics and Ontology   29
    3.1   Introduction   29
    3.2   Ontology..   30
        3.2.1   What is an Ontology........................   30
        3.2.2   Generic Ontologies and Specific Ontologies........   31
    3.3   The Ontology Argument   32
    3.4   Ontology Modelling Notation.........................   35
    3.5   Purposes for Which Ontologies are Being Used   39
        3.5.1   Strong and Unambiguous Communication
                Mechanism   40
        3.5.2   Ontology Mediated Information Access...........   41
        3.5.3   Ontology and Semantic Web Services...........   42
        3.5.4   Ontology Based Multi Agent Systems...........   46
    3.6   Ontology Modelling and Representation   46
    3.7   Differentiating Conceptual Modelling for Data Modelling,
        Knowledge Modelling and Ontology Modelling
        and a Notation for Ontology Modelling.................   48
    3.8   W3C—The Strong Metadata Modeling Promoter   52
    3.9   The Web is an Information Treasure Trove   53
    3.10   Some Insight into RDF and OWL.....................   54
    3.11   Transformation of Markup Languages   61
    3.12   OWL Language   63
    3.13   Recapitulation   64
    Appendix 1.......................................   65
    Appendix 2.......................................   69
    References...   74

4   Ontology for Traditional Chinese Medicine (TCM)   77
    4.1   Introduction   77
    4.2   Usefulness of Ontology in TCM.......................   77
    4.3   Semantic Aliasing...................................   79
    4.4   Choice of Modeling Tools............................   83
    4.5   The Realm of Metadata Modeling.....................   89

4.6   Enterprise TCM Ontology Core   90
4.7   Cross-Layer Onto-Core Semantic Transitivity (COST).......   93
4.8   COST Check Anytime and Anywhere...................   95
4.9   Recapitulation   97
References...   97

5   **Ontology Driven System Generation and Remote Installation**   99
5.1   Introduction...................................   99
5.2   The Mobile-Clinic Experience Unveils the Importance
       of Ontological Adherence   99
5.3   Provision of Standard Diagnosis and Prescription   102
5.4   Error-Free System Customization by the Meta-Interface
       (MI) Concept..................................   105
5.5   Automatic Remote Web-Based Installation...............   109
5.6   Recapitulation   113
References...   116

6   **Ontology Evolution and the Living TCM Ontology**   117
6.1   Introduction...................................   117
6.2   "Living/Live" Onto-core to Support On-line Evolution   118
6.3   Knowledge and Experience Absorption   120
6.4   Enablement of Easy Knowledge Reabsorption
       and Evolution..................................   123
       6.4.1   "Living Ontology" Aids Knowledge Absorption
                and Evolution...........................   123
6.5   Coherent Consensus-Certified Knowledge Engineering   126
6.6   Recapitulation   128
References...   128

7   **TCM Telemedicine Infrastructure**   129
7.1   Introduction...................................   129
7.2   Performance Modelling of the Pervasive TCM
       Telemedicine Infrastructure on the Mobile Internet   129
7.3   Realization Example   133
7.4   Recapitulation   136
References...   136

8   **Recapitulation and Future Directions**....................   137
8.1   Introduction...................................   137
8.2   Recapitulation   137
8.3   Future Work   139
       8.3.1   Collaborative Multi Agent Recommender Systems ...   139
       8.3.2   Integrative Medicine   140

        8.3.3   Cloud Computing for TCM Telemedicine   141
        8.3.4   Cyber Physical Systems and the Internet of Things
                 for TCM Telemedicine   143
    8.4   Conclusion.   151
    References.   151

About the Authors

Prof. Allan K.Y. Wong was Assistant Professor and Undergraduate Course Leader in The Department of Computing, The Hong Kong Polytechnic University. Allan received PolyU Technology and Consultancy Company Limited Highest Growth Consultant Award (Merit) for consultancy activities in 2008. He was a listed Chinese medicine practitioner registered in the Chinese Medicine Council of Hong Kong and was a permanent member and past executive of the Kowloon (Hong Kong) Chinese Herbalists Association. Allan is the co-author of the books "Streetwise Guide: Chinese Herbal Medicine" ISBN-13: 978-1891688010 and co-author of the book "Harnessing the Service Roundtrip Time over the Internet to Support Time-Critical Applications: Concepts, Techniques and Cases" ISBN:1-60021-604-8.

Dr. Jackei H.K. Wong is the co-founder and Chief Information Officer of Herb-Miners Informatics Limited. Jackei is the honorary chairman and life member of the Association of Hong Kong and Kowloon Practitioners of Chinese Medicine Limited—Chinese Medical Research Institute. He received the Ph.D. degree at the Hong Kong Polytechnic University in 2010. Jackei has over 8 years' experience in Research and Development, and more than 20 refereed journals and conference publications. His research interests include data mining, TCM ontology, cloud computing, big data analysis and information retrieval.

Dr. Wilfred W.K. Lin is the co-founder and Chief Research Officer of HerbMiners Informatics Limited. Wilfred is the honorary chairman and life member of the Association of Hong Kong and Kowloon Practitioners of Chinese Medicine Limited—Chinese Medical Research Institute. He received the Ph.D. degree at the Hong Kong Polytechnic University in 2005 and also received the Gold Silk Ball Award, The People's Government of Guangxi Zhuang Autonomous Region in 2010. Wilfred has over 14 years' experience in Research and Development, co-authored two textbooks and more than 60 refereed journals and conference publications. His research interests include data mining, TCM ontology, cloud computing, big data analysis and information retrieval.

Prof. Tharam S. Dillon has published more than 800 papers in international conferences and journals, ten authored books and six edited books. His work has over 8,500 citations and he has an H-Index of 43 (source Google Scholar). His research interests include Cyber Physical Systems, Data mining, Neural Networks, Web semantics, ontologies, Internet computing, cloud computing, hybrid neuro-symbolic systems, software engineering, database systems and power systems computation. Prof. Dillon is a Life Fellow of the IEEE (USA). Prof. Dillon is a Fellow of ACS and IEAust. He has a widely known international reputation. He is Editor-in-Chief of three international journals, namely the International Journal of Computer Systems Science and Engineering, the International Journal of Electric Power and Energy Systems, and the International Journal of Engineering Intelligent Systems. He is a member of several international technical committees and working groups and was the chairman of the International CIGRE Task Force 38-06-02 on Expert Systems for Monitoring and Alarm Processing in Control Centres. He is also a member of IFIP Working Group 2.6 on Knowledge and Data Semantics.

Prof. Elizabeth J. Chang is Professor and Canberra Fellow in the School of Business, the University of New South Wales at the Australian Defence Force Academy. Her current research focuses on Defence Force Logistics; Military Transport Systems, Ambient Security, Cyber-Physical Logistics Infrastructure and Networks; Trust and Risks, Emergency Situation Awareness; Virtual Collaborative Logistics and underlying technologies including data intelligence and real time big data analytics. She is the Chair elect for the IEEE IES Technical Committee on Industrial Informatics (2014–2015) where she will provide leadership in this area in the world by attracting top talent and researchers from around the world to help define the future research directions. She is also an Associate Editor for IEEE Transactions on Industrial Electronics (since 2007) and Guest Editor on IEEE Transactions on Industrial Informatics (since 2005), Co-editor in chief for International Journal on Engineering Intelligent Systems. She is a member of Council of Supply Chain Management Professionals, honorary member of the Australian Logistics and Supply Chain Society, Senior Member of IEEE and she was honoured to be Technical Chair or General chair for over 20 International and IEEE Conferences.

Chapter 1
Telemedicine and Knowledge Representation for Traditional Chinese Medicine

1.1 Traditional Chinese Medicine and a Consensus Certified Knowledge Base

The knowledge of Traditional Chinese Medicine (TCM) has been in existence for more than 3,000 years. However, TCM was practised in various forms according to the constraints imposed by the different geographical and environmental conditions. Due to transportation difficulties, political turmoil, language barriers and various reasons at that time, the chance of exchanging medical knowledge and clinical experience was limited. This ability to exchange knowledge was greatly enhanced only much later in the Qin dynasty (a few centuries BC) that united China into a single empire with a standard writing system, improved road conditions and transportation means. This was the prelude to the first successful *Yellow Emperor's Canon of Internal Medicine* (*Huang Di Nei Jing*), which is still the ultimate TCM reference today. Practically, this Canon compiled medical knowledge and clinical experience within the Qin territory into a single entity to facilitate education, training and transmission of TCM expertise.

In the early days before the Qin dynasty, as well in remote areas until fairly recently, clinical experiences were recorded in different ways by different communities, such as oracle bones/shells, chanting, inscriptions and other artefacts. As time passed, this recorded medical information has been gradually refined, carefully and painstakingly, to eventually constitute more than 5,000 medical works in extant. The process of TCM knowledge refinement has been supported by both civilian and governmental effort over time. As time progressed, useful herbal ingredients, which include plant parts, minerals and animal matter, have been added and incorporated into the conceptual TCM pharmacopoeia.

In the olden days, a TCM practitioner was usually conversant with a combination of several areas of professional knowledge to a varying degree including internal medicine, nutrition, surgery, bone setting and veterinary medicine. As knowledge and experience has been accumulating, TCM required more sophisticated specialization

© Springer-Verlag Berlin Heidelberg 2015
A.K.Y. Wong et al., *Semantically Based Clinical TCM Telemedicine Systems*,
Studies in Computational Intelligence 587, DOI 10.1007/978-3-662-46024-5_1

in a specific area, for example, gynaecology in internal medicine. This increase in specialization requirements means reduction in the knowledge of other medical faculties such as bone-setting and veterinary medicine. Modern TCM training and clinical practice also include some techniques from Western medicine. Some examples include the use of X-rays, syringe-based injection and laboratory tests.

Whilst Traditional Chinese Medicine (TCM) has been widely used for many centuries in China, more recently one has seen TCM get a wider world wide adoption. Thus, in western countries which were previously dominated by Allopathic medicine, one often sees TCM practitioners conducting successful practices. Another emerging trend has been the adoption of some elements of TCM in their practice by doctors trained in the Western Allopathic Medical Tradition. Thus, we see these doctors use acupuncture and TCM herbs along with the allopathic drugs. This tendency is expected to grow in the future as information and knowledge about TCM becomes more widespread.

Many of these trends in the use of TCM will be aided by the use of a uniform vocabulary and an agreed consensus on the body of knowledge in TCM. This motivates us in this book to capture the underlying clinical TCM Body of Knowledge and practices in a computer based representation. This computer based representation has a semantic basis in which the focus is on the meaning of the knowledge rather than the syntactic format of its representation. We also organize the representation of the knowledge to make it more coherent and easily understandable by both humans and computers. Using this approach it makes the knowledge more readily searchable and queried. We utilize an ontology for doing this. Ontologies are discussed more fully in Chap. 3 and their use for representing TCM knowledge is discussed in Chap. 4. Here it is sufficient to understand that the ontology contains consensus certified knowledge capturing concepts and relationships.

1.2 Traditional Chinese Medicine and Telemedicine

In order to make this knowledge actionable and widely distributed to practitioners, it is necessary to develop a framework that will permit clinics at sites geographically remote from the server where the ontology is stored to access this knowledge. It would also be valuable for mobile clinics to receive support from this semantic representation of TCM knowledge. A framework that provides this is the Telemedicine framework. Let us begin by exploring the Telemedicine framework.

1.2.1 What is Telemedicine?

One of the earliest definitions of the notion of Telemedicine is given in the publication [Lacroix99]. The basic requirement is to make use of the Internet to deliver medical care to every corner of the world. In this light any web-based medical system, independent of its size, has at least some telemedicine capability.

Telemedicine systems can be broadly divided into different types with respect to their functions and goals as follows:

(a)   Curative systems—medical practitioners use the system to achieve the diagnosis and treatment goals.
(b)   Consultative systems—through the system interface the user can obtain needed information, such as information about named patent drugs, and addresses/expertise of medical practitioners in the region/vicinity.
(c)   Medical information management systems in terms of data storage and retrieval (e.g. medical images).
(d)   Decision support systems—this happens in various forms, for example, the physician, who is using a telemedicine system (e.g. the PuraPharm's D/P (diagnosis/prescription) system in a mobile clinic [JWong09c] may import biometric reports to aid the diagnostic decision/precision as shown by Fig. 1.1.

The telemedicine domain consists of different distinctive and yet intertwined areas such as the following:

1.   Knowledge consultation
2.   Curative aspects
3.   Training by e-learning
4.   Management and control
5.   Efficient and reliable Information Communication Technology (ICT) support
6.   Explicit semantics

These are discussed in turn below.

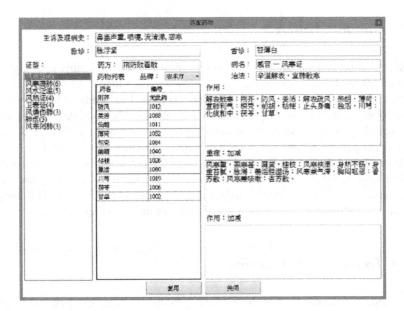

Fig. 1.1 Imported information to aid diagnosis

1.2.2 Knowledge Consultation

The aim is to let people including laymen and registered medical personnel consult and verify knowledge if necessary from the knowledge base. Yet, a knowledge base can be general purpose and similar to a dictionary in this sense. It can also be there to help experts to clarify doubts due to multi-representations owing to disparate national or regional conceptions of a medical phenomenon. A typical example in the Western/allopathic medicine area is the Unified Medical Language System (UMLS) [UMLS], which was developed by the USA National Library of Medicine to resolve the differences in Western/allopathic clinical terminology due to regional and/or national disparities. The UMLS is ontology-based. Another ontology based system is the disease and treatment ontology for Western Allopathic Medicine [Hadzic05, Hadzic10]. By its nature the UMLS is not for frontline clinical application to allow computer-aided diagnosis and treatment in contrast to the Nong's Traditional Chinese Medicine (TCM) telemedicine mobile clinic (MC) system discussed later. The UMLS is consultative in nature. That is, it is not a clinical system but a consultation setup that people can interact with to sort out terminology problems. Therefore, its aim is to provide an interactive learning, reference, and bridging mechanism for knowledge gaps in a global sense. For example, in conventional/Western/allopathic medicine different countries may have different definitions for an observed phenomenon. In order to resolve the similarity and differences of various definitions, as well as language peculiarities on a global scale, meta-thesauri can serve as an effective means as shown by the *Unified Medical Language System* (UMLS) [UMLS].

1.2.3 Curative Aspects

In this area the systems are for frontline diagnosis/prescription purposes. A good example of such a system is the Nong's Traditional Chinese Medicine (TCM) telemedicine mobile clinic (MC) system The mobile clinic (MC) system [JWong09c] is a decision support system that suggests the possible illnesses and corresponding prescriptions with respect to a given set of symptoms that are already encoded as part of the entities in the supporting TCM ontology—called the local TCM ontology core (or simply TCM onto-core). The physician has to decide on the exact illness and prescription because he/she is assigned this task and carries the legal liability associated with the assignment. As is the case for the UMLS architecture, the ontological information is contained in the meta-thesaurus.

1.2.4 Training by E-Learning

This helps train/retrain/update the medical personnel so that can carry out their duties accurately with the best and contemporary skills. At the professional level the knowledge base for the training/retraining purpose should at least be a semantic group or a subset of the conceptual subsumption hierarchy.

1.2.5 Management and Control

This functional module makes a telemedicine system have a "national" purpose in that it provides the medical statistics that feed into national medical policy especially in disease prevention and control. Information from medical cases provides disease/drug use profiles/statistics for the government/operator to dynamically re-adjust their management/control. At the enterprise level it helps efficient workflow scheduling and formulation of optimal inventory and/or manufacturing strategies for maximum financial benefit. For the PuraPharm Group, a local reputable pharmaceutical manufacturer in the Hong Kong SAR, such information represents an extra dimension—drug manufacturing strategy alignment. This alignment helps the company reap the maximum financial benefit from the statistics by setting up optimal seasonal manufacturing logistics.

1.2.6 Efficient and Reliable Information Communication Technology (ICT) Support

This implies two things: (a) the communication in the form of client/server message passing which should have a short service roundtrip time (RTT); and (b) bug free software support.

1.2.7 Explicit Semantics

If a single statement consisting of a string pattern can have different interpretations for different people with different perspectives, then the semantics of this string is considered implicit. This is similar to deciphering the embedded logic in a given program without its original high-level specification. The logical representation can vary from one interpreter to another. For example, the hierarchy represented in the Unified Modeling Language (UML) style in Fig. 1.2 can result in ambiguous interpretations (i.e. semantics) from different people for the "logical points" a and b, which can be logically AND or OR; vice versa; or EXCLUSIVE OR, leading to unexpected results. For curative medicine, this kind of logical freedom is disadvantageous to the patients. For this reason the semantics in the ontology *must be explicitly defined* by the principle of "one meaning for every semantic path".

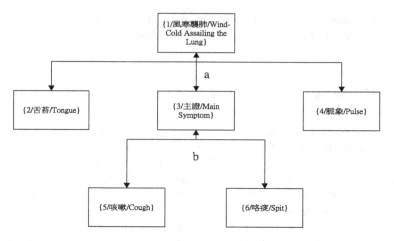

Fig. 1.2 Implicit logical representation—implicit semantics (bilingual)

The 3-dimensional subsumption hierarchy in Fig. 1.3 contains many *operations or semantic paths* (e.g. {3,5,8} and {3,6,9}). Yet, from a 2-dimensional viewpoint Fig. 1.2 is simply a network representation of many possible operational paths (i.e. traversal paths) between any two points. To create an operational ontology-based system (with a mini-ontology) out of this tree, it is necessary to elaborate this 2-dimensional view into a 3-dimensional one. Then, the focus is represented by the chosen "lead", which in reality is the first point where the parsing mechanism begins to process. For example, if node 1 is the chosen lead for parsing in Fig. 1.3, then the possible 14 semantic paths for the 3-dimensional subsumption hierarchy are the following: {1,2}; {1,3}; {1,3,5}; {1,3,5,8}; {1,3,6}; {1,3,6,9}; {1,3,6,10}; {1,4}; {1,4,7}; {1,4,7,6}; {1,4,7,6,9}; and {1,4,7,6,10}. If every semantic path is supported by only a single dedicated software module/object, then the meanings of the set of semantic paths (represented by the equal number of software modules or objects) form the lexicon for this particular system. As a result, the system always gives a clear, consistent and unambiguous (i.c. **_explict_**) answer to every query,

Fig. 1.3 Semantic paths in a 3-dimensional semantic subsumption hierarchy

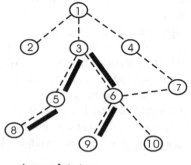

A complete tree

which is another form of a semantic path in the lexicon. Although the semantic paths in the lexicon are explicit, every query is constructed "implicitly" or with user-transparency according to the input sequence of the atomic elements. In fact, the semantic paths can be further classified into more specific semantic groups for various goals, similar in fashion to the conceptual UMLS framework.

1.3 Automatic System Generation and Evolution of the TCM Knowledge

In order to make the system practically usable, an important issue that has to be addressed is the development of an approach for system generation for each user or group of users that commits effectively to the ontology. To do this, we utilize an automatic system generation approach that is ontology driven. This approach is necessary to retain the relevant portions of the ontology and create alignment within the reasoning pathways and the user interface on each local implementation of the software necessary to access the ontology. We give an overview of this Automatic System Generation Approach in Sect. 1.5 and give a full discussion of it in Chap. 5.

In the last two sections, we considered the need for a semantic representation of knowledge of TCM within a computer system and the mechanisms for providing access to this from remote, distributed sites and mobile clinics.

The discussion in Sect. 1.1 emphasized the need for capturing the TCM knowledge within a consensus certified knowledge base that utilized a common vocabulary and concepts and terms. This representation captures the TCM knowledge at a particular point in time. However, we know that knowledge in the Allopathic Western Medicine is constantly growing. Similarly in Traditional Chinese Medicine, knowledge is constantly being generated as a result of new insights arising from research, clinical practice, experience and observation by TCM practitioners. In order to cater for this growing and evolving knowledge in the field, we need mechanisms for evolving this consensus certified knowledge in a semi automatic fashion. In Sect. 1.4.1 we give an overview and in Chap. 6, we discuss the framework for such ontology evolution [JWong09d].

1.4 Major Aspects of the Ontology Base TCM Telemedicine System

This book is focused on the scientific and engineering issues that underpin the building of a semantically-based clinical TCM telemedicine system successfully. It will address the following issues to a varying degree: (a) the meaning of telemedicine which we discussed in Sect. 1.2 of this chapter, (b) the TCM ambit, (c) usefulness of ontology in the building of computer-aided TCM systems,

(d) choice of the tool for modeling the ontology blueprint layout, (e) TCM tele-medicine infrastructure and mobile clinics, (f) ontology myth and conceptualiza-tion, how telemedicine system building can be automated with quality assurance, and (g) how a telemedicine prototype can be and deployed over the web.

This requires that we address the following aspects:

(a) Ontology modelling
(b) Ontology implementation tool
(c) Internet capability
(d) Architecture and cross-layer logical transitivity
(e) Automatic system generation
(f) Pervasive support
(g) Ontology evolution

1.4.1 Ontology Modelling

The design of the system begins with the ontology model blueprint layout followed by consensus certification. The ontology includes the whole or part of the for-malisms and knowledge in the relevant domain. In this sense, an ontology-based system is data/knowledge oriented. The ontology modelling notation given in Sect. 3.3 of Chap. 3 and Appendix 1 is for expressing the ontology model. This model should be understandable both by TCM domain experts and system devel-opers so as to facilitate evaluation and critiquing of the ontology by the domain experts for correctness and completeness.

1.4.2 Ontology Implementation Tool

The tool is usually a high level language, which can relate all the concepts in the ontology into a logical subsumption hierarchy. The ontology modelling blueprint is mainly for human understanding, and the embedded subsumption hierarchy should be translated meticulously into the corresponding semantic net for machine understanding/processing/execution. Therefore, it is necessary to choose a tool that has the support of ontology model blueprint-to-semantic-net translation. It is better for the conversion process to be automatic [JWong08b]. In this light, the languages (or metadata models/systems) proposed by W3C (World Wide Web Consortium) [W3Ca, W3Cb], namely, Extensible Mark-up Language (XML), Resource Description Framework (RDF), and Web Ontology Language (OWL) are good choices, for they have widespread automatic translation support.

1.4.3 Internet Capability

Telemedicine relies on the Internet to achieve different goals on the web. For example, the telemedicine system may send out miners to search the web for necessary information to support the system's ontology evolution—the concept of a living ontology [JWong08a]. This is well exemplified by the 2nd generation of the PuraPharm D/P (diagnosis/prescription) telemedicine system that supports Yan Oi Tong (YOT) mobile clinics in Hong Kong. These vehicle-based mobile clinics have been treating thousands of patients weekly in the past few years.

1.4.4 Architecture and Cross-layer Logical Transitivity

A practical telemedicine system should have a 3-layer architecture. These three layers are as follows:

- Bottom Layer—The bottom layer is the knowledge/database that embeds the subsumption hierarchy that represents the logical relationships among the physical data items/entities included in the consensus-certified ontology.
- Middle Layer—This subsumption hierarchy is also realized in the middle layer as the semantic net for machine understanding and execution.
- Top Layer—The top layer is the query system that implements the ontology for user understanding and manipulation.

The user enters a query or command via the system interface. This query is translated by the middle layer into the form understood by the semantic net, which executes the command and fetches the information for the user as the response.

The three layers are logically clones of one another, and therefore they should have cross-layer semantic transitivity. With this transitivity any entity in any layer should have corresponding representations in the other two layers. This three-layer architecture and cross layer logical transitivity are explained more fully in Chap. 4. It is useful here to compare our proposed architecture for the TCM Curative and Decision Support System with the 3-layer architecture of the UMLS consultation system.

The UMLS is ontology-based and also has three distinctive layers (Fig. 1.4): (i) the modularized query system (the modules are semantic groups) at the top level, (ii) the middle logical semantic-net layer, which was constructed from the semantics embedded in the information of the bottom ontological layer, and (iii) the bottom ontology is integrated by nature and normally has a subsumption hierarchy of various sub-ontologies of different origins [Gruber93a, Gruber93b, Gyurino95].

There is, therefore, some similarity between the overall structures of the two systems even though one is used for Curative and Decision Support Purposes whilst another one is used as a consultation system.

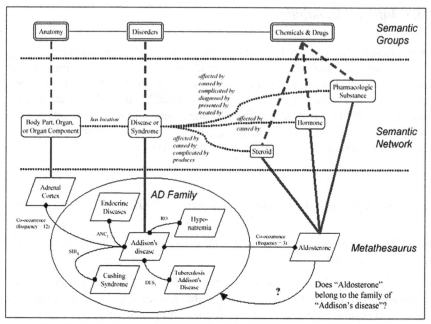

Overview of the methodology applied to the relationships of "Aldosterone" to "Addison's disease"

Fig. 1.4 The 3-layer UMLS hierarchy [UMLS]

1.4.5 Automatic System Generation

Cross-layer semantic transitivity can be achieved correctly by automatic system generation or customization (ASG/C). This approach is, in fact, a new software engineering paradigm, which requires the user to provide the ontology blueprint layout. With support of the master ontology, where the ontology specification is either a part or the whole of it, the ASG/C mechanism generates/customizes the final ontology-based system in one shot [JWong08a].

1.4.6 Pervasive Support

A telemedicine system needs the support of a wireless-based pervasive computing infrastructure (PCI), which maintains the smart spaces for the collaborating systems. In the PuraPharm mobile-clinics environment, the collaborating systems are the mobile clinics. The essence of the PCI support is better explained by using the successful PuraPharm's mobile-clinic (MC) based telemedicine D/P (diagnosis/ prescription) system depicted in Fig. 1.5. The PCI maintains the smart spaces, which is each occupied by a mobile clinic. The mobile clinic then communicates

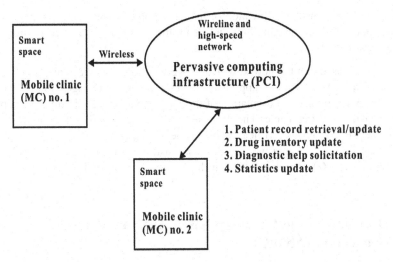

Fig. 1.5 A PuraPharm's pervasive MC-based telemedicine D/P system

with the central system, as well as its peers, via the wireless means provided by the PCI. The MC operation is semi-autonomous because the physician can treat the patient at the spot, but the case history of the patient may have to be downloaded from the central computer that runs the fast network. The MC has to inform the central system of its updated local drug inventory. The central system also collects the necessary MC statistics on-line for proactive planning and action. If the MC physician needs help in the diagnostic process, the central system would solicit the relevant information from other friendly sites via the Internet.

1.4.7 Ontology Evolution Approach

It is important that the TCM ontology does not become frozen and outdated but is able to take into account the new knowledge and insights that are being generated as time passes. The TCM ontology should be able to absorb information from every fresh case into the "master" ontology as new knowledge. In this light, this master ontology is a living and evolving system. Hence, it is clear that there is a need for a framework of ontology evolution for the TCM ontology so that it reflects the new knowledge and insights. In this book, if any ontology is the basis for new rounds of consensus certifications, it is the master ontology, independent of its functional, domain, industrial or enterprise nature.

To achieve ontology evolution, we need to:

- Ascertain the new knowledge.
- Represent this potential new knowledge temporarily in a form compatible with Ontology.

- Carryout Consensus Certification of this new potential new knowledge.
- Enhancing the Master Ontology only with the Consensus Certified portions of the new knowledge.

In order to ascertain the new knowledge, we will utilize a text mining approach. The Data and Text Mining approach suggests potential changes to the TCM ontology. A temporary representation of these potential changes is stored in a part of the Master Aliasing Table. The proposed potential changes to the ontology are then subject to consensus certification by a panel of TCM Domain experts, and only those changes that are approved by this consensus certification are then included into the master TCM ontology through the Master Aliasing Table.

1.5 Overview of the Ontology-Based Automatic System Generation (ASG/C)

It is useful to provide an overview of the ontology-based automatic system generation here so that the reader can get a better appreciation of the approach. The details of the ASG/C process will be explained later in the relevant sections of Chap. 5.

The 3-layer architecture of the TCM System sheds light on how a practical ontology-based system should be built based on the following arguments:

(a) If the bottom ontological layer is the "required" knowledge by consensus certification, then the system created for the specification provided by a semantic group (top layer) only needs to be supported by the relevant portion, which is part of the master ontology. This portion, in effect, is isolated as the "local" ontology for the target system as specified. This isolation process is basically customization.

(b) If the specification by a semantic group is logically correct, then the corresponding error-free target system can be customized in one shot by using an appropriate automatic mechanism such as the *Enterprise Ontology Driven Information System Development* (EOD-ISD) paradigm [JWong08a]. The customization automation cuts the development costs and ensures customer satisfaction by its short development cycle.

(c) If the "total" ontological knowledge could be drawn as a network or DOM (*document object model—a synonym of the W3C for semantic net*) tree, the isolated "local" ontology for the target system should have its local parser to work on it. The parser finds the answer for the query $Q\{p_1, p_2\}$ at the syntactic semantic group level (or query level) by inference. It traces out the unique operation or semantic path in the DOM tree or semantic net in a suitable manner for the input parameter set. Machine processing in the ontological context is parsing.

From the literature, the only software engineering paradigm that can support the ASG/C process is the *enterprise ontology-driven information system development* (EOD-ISD) [JWong08a]. The core idea of this paradigm is to generate cognate system variants from the same TCM onto-core master automatically. For example, all the PuraPharm's D/P systems are customized from the proprietary master/ enterprise TCM onto-core by applying the EOD-ISD paradigm. Similar to the UMLS, a D/P system always has three layers: (i) the bottom layer—the portion of the consensus-certified master ontology known as the local onto-core for the target system; (ii) the middle parsing mechanism that works with the semantic sub-sumption hierarchy (i.e. semantic net) embedded in the local onto-core; and (iii) the query system that enables the user to interact with the system.

As shown in Fig. 1.6, which is the EOD-ISD overview, the first step in the EOD-ISD paradigm is to construct an iconic specification. This specification is made up of icons, which are either user-defined or standard ones selected from the pro-prietary library of predefined icons. Every icon, which represents a unique semantic path (e.g. {3,5,8}) of Fig. 1.3, is defined by two parts: the graphical representation, and its unique supporting software object/module that implements the semantic path and is therefore functionally distinctive.

In Fig. 1.7 the graphical icon is encircled on the right-hand side and its corre-sponding semantic/operational path is encircled on the left. They form the unique pair, either defined by the user or as a predefined couple stored in the master library of icons. In the first step of the EOD-ISD based automatic system generation process, the user provides the iconic or meta-interface (MI) specification made up of the set of selected icons. The EOD-ISD generator combines all the supporting semantic net modules (similar to the left-hand encirclement in Fig. 1.6) to construct the local system onto-core for the target system. This customized local onto-core is

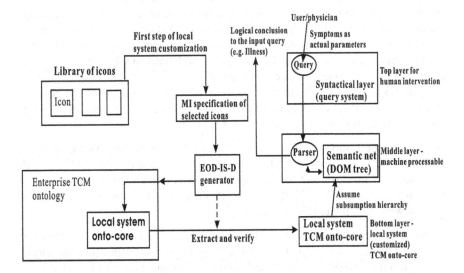

Fig. 1.6 The EOD-ISD approach overview

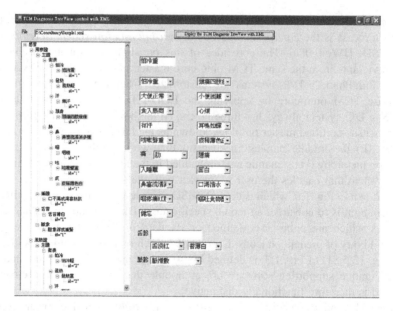

Fig. 1.7 Supporting semantic and the corresponding icon

basically a specified extraction of the relevant semantic paths from the master enterprise ontology. Considering from a W3C viewpoint, the local onto-core is a sub-tree of the master DOM tree. From the specified onto-core extraction, the corresponding semantic net is created with the standard parser inserted. Finally the query system is constructed to represent the semantic net for human understanding. The appearance of the query system interface is basically a mosaic of all the selected graphical icons. The semantic net can be implemented in any programming languages (e.g. Visual Basic for web application i.e. VB.net). The implementation in the form of a software object/module is called the component template (CT). The modular semantic net (as depicted in the left encirclement in Chinese of Fig. 1.7) can be expressed/encoded in different languages.

Figure 1.8 is the query interface of a real-life D/P system operated by the Nong's company. This D/P system is generated from an icon specification consisting of the following (its English version is shown in Fig. 1.9):

(a) Component Template CT (I) is the "control bar", which shows the specific functions. In this case, the "diagnosis and prescription or D/P (診治)" icon/ function is invoked, and the corresponding meta-interface is displayed.

(b) Component Template CT (II) is the "D/P" meta-interface, which has nested the following Component Templates (CTs):

    (i) Component Template CT (III) records the currently observed symptoms (症候群), which can be "**inferred** *by the system*" from the laboratory results (實驗室-化驗報告)and *key-in* data by the physician (e.g. 梁偉文)

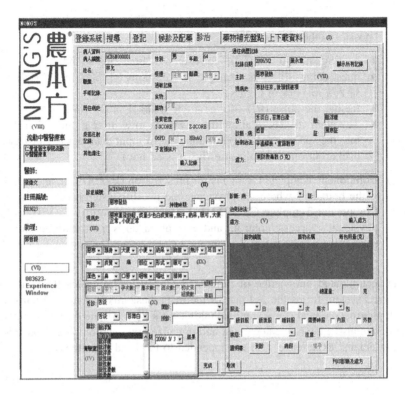

Fig. 1.8 Identification of iconic or meta-interface regions

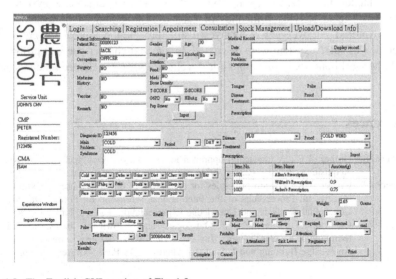

Fig. 1.9 The English GUI version of Fig. 1.8

based on the four principles (四診) {seeing (望)—for example "舌診" and "possibly others—"皮/甲診",

- hearing-smell-touch (聞)—for example "breathing sound",
- questioning (問)—for example 10 questions [十問歌 in CT (IX) and 婦人尤問月事 in CT (X)],
- feeling the pulse (切)—for example (脈診)} in CT (IV)}.
- The alternative is to allow the physician to write (e.g. through Tablet) into the space in CT (III) but this kind of input data lacks "consensus" backup in ontological sense (i.e. it is ad hoc).

(ii) Component Template CT (V) is for prescription (處方/配藥), and CT (V) is the boundary where the physician and the dispenser/pharmacist meet.

(iii) Component Template CT (VII) is the patient's record; CT (VIII) is the physician's access control, and the physician's personal/accumulated experience can be referred to through Component Template CT (VI).

The accumulated knowledge of different Component Templates (CTs) in the customized system forms the 3rd part of the meta-thesaurus [the other 2 parts are formal: pharmacological (藥理) and pathological (病理)]. All the data in the meta-interface are also captured, categorized and organized into sub-ontology constructs (e.g. physicians' experience) that are appended to the local meta-thesaurus.

1.6 Recapitulation

In this chapter, the need for a semantically based TCM telemedicine system was examined. The underlying principles of such a TCM telemedicine system were briefly explored. An overview of its layered structure and the approach to automatic generation of such a system were discussed. In the next chapter, we will probe into the TCM world and its implications for developing a TCM telemedicine system.

References

[Gruber93a] Gruber, T.R.: A translation approach to portable ontology specification. Knowl. Acquisition 5(2), 199–220 (1993)
[Gruber93b] Gruber, T.R.: Toward principles for the design of ontologies used for knowledge sharing. In: Proceedings of the International Workshop on Formal Ontology in Conceptual Analysis and Knowledge Representation, Padova, Italy, 17 Mar 1993
[Guarino95] Guarino, N., Giaretta, P.: Ontologies and knowledge bases: towards a terminological clarification. In: Towards Very Large Knowledge Bases: Knowledge Building and Knowledge Sharing, IOS Press, Amsterdam, pp. 25–32 (1995)

[Hadzic05]   Hadzic, M., Chang, E.: Medical ontologies to support human disease research and control. Int. J. Web Grid Serv. **1**(2), 139–150 (2005)

[Hadzic10]   Hadzic, M., Wongthongtham, P., Dillon, T., Chang, E.: Ontology-Based Multi-Agent Systems. Springer Publications, Germany, 274 p (2010). ISBN 978-3-642-01903-6

[Lacroix99]   Lacroix, A., Lareng, L., Rossignol, G., Padeken, D., Bracale, M., Ogushi, Y., Wootton, R., Sanders, J., Preost, S., McDonald, I.: G-7 global healthcare applications sub-project 4, international concerted action on collaboration in telemedicine. http://www.atmeda.org/ICOT/finalReport.G8SP.4 (1999). Accessed 10 Jun 2005

[UMLS]   UMLS: http://umls.nlm.nih.gov/

[W3Ca]   W3C: Ontology definition MetaModel. http://www.omg.org/docs/ad/05-08-01.pdf (2005). Accessed 16 Sept 2005

[W3Cb]   W3C: Web service architecture (working paper). http://www.w3.org/TR/ws-arch/

[JWong09d]   Wong, J.H.K.: Web-based data mining and discovery of useful herbal ingredients (WD^{2}UHI). PhD thesis, Department of Computing, Hong Kong Polytechnic University (2009)

[JWong08a]   Wong, J.H.K., Dillon, T.S., Wong, A.K.Y., Lin, W.W.K.: Text mining for real-time ontology evolution. In: Data Mining for Business Applications, Springer, pp. 143–150 (2008). ISBN 978-0-387-79419-8

[JWong08b]   Wong, J.H.K., Lin, W.W.K., Wong, A.K.Y., Dillon, T.S.: An ontology supported meta-interface for the development and installation of customized web-based telemedicine systems. In: Proceedings of the 6th IFIP Workshop on Software Technologies for Future Embedded and Ubiquitous Systems (SEUS), Capri Island, Italy, 1–3 Oct 2008

[JWong09c]   Wong, J.H.K., Lin, W.W.K., Wong, A.K.Y., Dillon, T.S.: TCM (Traditional Chinese Medicine) telemedicine with enterprise ontology support—a form of consensus-certified collective human intelligence. In: Proceedings of the International Conference on Industrial Technology (ICIT), Monash University, Victoria, Australia, 10–13 Feb 2009

Chapter 2
The TCM Ambit

2.1 The Evolution of Traditional Chinese Medicine

As noted in Chap. 1, the use of Traditional Chinese Medicine (TCM) has been around for more than 3,000 years. In its early period, due to difficulties of exchanging medical knowledge and clinical experience, TCM was practiced in various forms often dictated by different geographical and environmental conditions. With the rise of the Qin Dynasty that united China into a single empire with a standard writing system, the ability to exchange knowledge was greatly facilitated. This led to the first successful *Yellow Emperor's Canon of Internal Medicine* (*Huang Di Nei Jing*), which remains an important TCM reference till today. This Canon comprises medical knowledge and clinical experience within the Qin territory.

As time passed, recorded medical and clinical information has been gradually refined, supported by both the civilian and governmental effort, and eventually constitutes more than 5,000 medical works. Useful herbal ingredients, which include plant parts, minerals and animal matter, have also been incorporated into the conceptual TCM pharmacopoeia.

Whilst earlier TCM practitioners were usually conversant with the broad combination of many areas of professional knowledge, TCM practitioners required more specialization in a specific area. This increase in specialization meant reduction in the knowledge of the areas. Modern TCM training and clinical practice also include incorporated techniques from Western medicine, including techniques such as use of X-rays, syringe-based injection and laboratory tests. It is a professional requirement that a TCM practitioner should have knowledge of nutrition to help patients recover from illnesses quicker and better. In TCM drug administration the base concept is that the continuum of food material can be divided into two basic categories: curative and health restoring. Yet, it is common that a health-restoring ingredient may become a prescribe-able main curative herb (e.g. Ren shen/Panax ginseng).

© Springer-Verlag Berlin Heidelberg 2015
A.K.Y. Wong et al., *Semantically Based Clinical TCM Telemedicine Systems*,
Studies in Computational Intelligence 587, DOI 10.1007/978-3-662-46024-5_2

TCM (Traditional Chinese Medicine) as we know it today includes several Canons as its foundation, including:

1. *The Yellow Emperor's Canon of Internal Medicine (Huang Di Nei Jing)*, which was formulated in the eighth century BC (circa 722 BC), is the earliest treatise in the field. It is still revered as the ultimate medical reference by many TCM practitioners. The *Nei Jing* is rich in its contents and includes human body anatomy, physiology, acupuncture, blood circulation and its relationship to breathing and heart/pulse rate.
2. *Shen Nong's Canon on Materia Medica (Shen Nong Ben Cao Jing)*, which was compiled by the Han Emperor's decree in the 1st century AD. This contains more than 800 commonly used herbs for medical treatment during that period.

The *Compendium of Materia Medica (Ben Cao Gang Mu)*, which was compiled by a reputable TCM practitioner in the 16th century, Li Shizhen. This records the usage of almost 2,000 herbal ingredients. It provides a much stronger pharmacological foundation than the *Shen Nong's Canon*, and it is still strongly adhered to in today's TCM practice. Many herbal ingredients and their clinical efficacy are increasingly included in the Western medicine pharmacopoeia. The well-known example is Artemisia (Qinghao), which is remarkably effective for treating malaria. In fact, in the People's Republic of China (PRC) many hospitals are "mixed" in nature, practising both TCM and Western medicine at the same time. Which expertise plays the lead role and is complemented by the other depends on the illness and the physical condition of the patient at the time. It is not uncommon that the medical team formed to treat a patient is made up of both TCM and Western medicine practitioners. This approach helps speed up the inclusion of herbal ingredients in the domain of Western pharmacopoeia. It is interesting to note that food and medicine are in the same continuum within the Compendium. This explains why TCM practitioners always try to maximize medicinal treatment by complementing it with strong suggestions of proper nutrition.

In the Ming (1368–1644) and Qing (1644–1840) Dynasties, TCM had advanced tremendously because of support from the government, especially in the areas of anatomy, etiology of disease, treating communicable illnesses and methodical applications of various herbal ingredients. As a result, a wide range of principles for diagnosis, therapies and principles for dispensing drugs were formalized to treat ailments in an easier and more standard way. This is well reflected by clinical TCM practice today.

2.2 Underlying Theory

The anatomy of the human body in the TCM view differs from the conventional biological concept. The main difference is the inclusion of the conceptual network of meridians and collaterals. The meridians associate with the corresponding organs such as the liver and the spleen. This organs-meridians association is verifiable from the point of view of acupuncture. The explanation of health maintenance is also different from the conventional physiology approach. In TCM, health is maintained if the Yin and the Yang in the body are balanced [Maciocia05]. The main task for the physician to treat a patient is to get rid of the excess (Yin or Yang) and supplement the deficiencies (Yin or Yang). If the human body is correctly balanced by Yin (material base) and Yang (metabolism), then the equilibrium brings about and maintains health. Therefore, the most important concept in TCM is to maintain this equilibrium by eliminating excesses and supplementing deficiencies. The metabolism consumes the material and converts it into the necessary vital energy flow (Qi) in the body, and we need proper nutrition to support the material base (Yin). TCM differs from Western medicine by stressing that every vital organ (e.g. liver) in our body has its own unique Qi characteristic. There are 12 conceptual organs all together, namely, (1) the solid Yin viscera: heart, liver, spleen, lung, kidney and "pericardium" (i.e. the layer of membranous tissue surrounding the heart), and (2) the hollow Yang bowels: small intestine, gall bladder, stomach, large intestine, urinary bladder (including the "female capsule"—i.e. reproductive system), and "triple warmers/burners" (i.e. the three body cavities, namely, (a) above the waist, (b) at the diaphragm and umbilicus, and (c) below the umbilicus). Every organ has its specific channel (technically called the Jing or meridian) for its Qi to flow through, and that is why our body has 12 organ-based Qi channels or meridians. The pattern of the Qi flow reflects the health condition of the organ. The Qi in the meridians interact to maintain our health or metabolic equilibrium via the smaller Qi ducts (technically called the Lok or collaterals). The 12 "organic" Qi channels, the numerous collaterals, and the two main Qi "highways" make up the complete Qi network of the body. Eventually, the Qi from the 12 meridians drains into the two main Qi "highways" to complete their flow cycles. The two main "highways" are the Ren meridian in the front of the main body and the Du meridian at the back. All the Yin Qi channels drain into the Ren meridian, whereas all the Yang ones drain into the Du meridian. The concept of Qi flow in the 14 meridians altogether provides the foundation for balancing the body's Yin and Yang to achieve health, and physiological and spiritual equilibrium. The spiritual part is a very important parameter of good health because it is achieved only when the body's Yin and Yang are balanced. The significance of this parameter is enshrined as a formal TCM axiom (formalism), namely, "If the Yin is sufficient and the Yang dynamics are stable, then a person will attain spiritual calmness". In the TCM domain consistent spiritual calmness is the gateway to longevity. If there is no blockage in the Qi flow of any kind, a person will be in the healthy state. To get rid of any Qi blockage, appropriate measure(s) such as herbal concoctions and acupuncture can be administered in a controlled and progressive manner. For this reason all the herbal ingredients are classified by two parameters, namely, their associations with the particular meridians/organs and their temperaments. The temperament includes heating, cooling, warming, "neutral" as far as the effect on the ambient body temperature is concerned; rising—bringing the curative drug effect upward to the body surface; sinking—bringing the curative drug effect downward deep inside the body; and conducting—bringing the curative drug effect to the desired spot, channel and organ. The details and meanings of herbal temperaments are formally documented in TCM Canons, and they will be explained later in this chapter.

2.3 TCM Diagnosis and Treatment

The process of diagnosis is based on the following formalisms, which have three broad categories, namely:

(a) The four steps:

  (i) Inspection—looking for apparent signs (e.g. acne/sores/ulceration/ eczema and tongue—its colour and texture), as well as usual visual conditions along the Qi meridians.

  (ii) Listening—searching for unusual sound uncontrollably made by the body part(s) (e.g. a hissing sound while the patient is breathing may indicate pneumonia or asthma).

  (iii) Questioning—asking questions about how the patient feels, his/her past sickness/treatment history, habits and dietary preferences (e.g. constipation? sudden surge/waves of fever and/or cold? insomnia? phlegm/sputum colour (e.g. yellow phlegm indicates possible inflammation in the lung)).

  (iv) Taking the patient's pulse based on the 8 principles and 4 basic pulsation guidelines—pulse waveforms have very specific and significant diagnostic meanings.

(b) The 8 principles for illness type identification:

  (i) Cold/heat types—these two principles differentiate the nature of the sickness being diagnosed; for example, anything of the anaemic nature is the cold type (and the treatment is to heat the body up) and any inflammation is the heat type (and the treatment is to "cool" the body, reducing the inflammation).

  (ii) Surface/internal types—the status of the sickness is surface because it has not impeded the core of the organ function (e.g. coughing/fever due to a flu is "surface" but pneumonia is "internal" because part(s) of the lung issue might have died).

  (iii) Deficient/excess types—the sickness is caused by Yin or Yang deficiency (e.g. blood loss) or excesses (e.g. indigestion due to gluttony); and Yin/ Yang types—if it is caused by material-based problems, then it is the Yin type (e.g. loss of blood), and if is caused by metabolic malfunctions/ blockages (e.g. gall/kidney stones), then it is the Yang type of problem.

(c) The 4 basic pulsation axioms: The four axiomatic guidelines, which help the physician to confirm the correctness in the interpretations of the 8 principles mentioned above, are as follows:

   (i) Floating—the pulse that can be felt on the standard/dedicated wrist-based positions is shallowly close to the skin surface; this usually indicates excessive heat rising from the body/organ(s), for dissipation purposes.
   (ii) Deep—the pulse can only be felt by pressing hard on the standard wrist-based points; this usually indicates slow/weak metabolism.
   (iii) Slow—slow pulsation means weak metabolism and Qi blockage.
   (iv) Fast—more serious inflammation normally produces rapid faster pulses of various forms. In fact, the 4 basic pulsation guidelines can be further differentiated during the pulse-taking process by recognizing the different additional tell-tale signs (e.g. a fast pulse in the shape of a sine wave (called "pearl-like" could mean lung inflammation for a man/woman, but further differentiation is needed to ensure it is not pregnancy (which typically manifests in the form of "pearl-like" pulses) for a woman).

The following illustrative medical case would help categorize the above diagnosis and herbal classification process differentiating the perspectives. In this case the symptoms obtained by the 4 axiomatic guidelines strongly indicate pneumonia at the early stage:

(a) Inspection—the patient coughs violently and needs to move his/her shoulder upward (i.e. to move the rib cage upward) to assist the coughing act. (It is worthwhile to mention here that modern TCM practice also inspects the X-ray images and other laboratory tests such as sputum analysis).
(b) Listening—the patient breathes with a hissing sound (one needs proper training to detect this phenomenon).
(c) Questioning—the answers from the patient reveal that the sputum is yellow and fever occurs in the late afternoon.
(d) Pulse—very fast "pearl-like" fast pulse that can be felt from the wrist surface.

The strong likelihood of pneumonia is further confirmed by applying the 8 axiomatic principles based on the diagnosis result:

(a) Heat type—inflammation in the lung.
(b) Internal type—part of the lung tissue could be severely injured.
(c) Deficient type—the severe injury of the lung tissue means damage (i.e. "loss") of the organ's material base causing Yin/Yang imbalance leading to inflammation and spurious heat (i.e. resultant surge of the Yang dynamics due to deficient Yin).
(d) Yin type—it is caused by material-based problems.

Different measures can be prescribed alone or in a combined manner (e.g. herbal concoctions and/or acupuncture) to treat the above case. The herbs in the concoction should ideally meet the following four aims: (i) the ***principal*** herb(s) should stop the lung inflammation; (ii) the ***adjuvant*** herb(s) should help repair the damaged lung tissue and neutralize the undesirable effect from the principal herb(s); (iii) the **_aux-iliary_** herb(s) helps catalyze, correct and accelerate the curative effects of the principal and adjuvant herbs and may also incite the sinking or rising of these effects; and (iv) the **_conductant_** (also known as **_messenger_**) herbs bring the overall curative effect to the sick organ and its Qi channel.

The prescription for treating the aforementioned pneumonia case example may consist of the following ingredients among other possible choices because it depends on the physician's experience and preference:

(a) The **_principal_** herbs: "Yu Xing Cao" (*Herba Houttuyniae*) and "Huang Qin" (*Radix Scutellariae*) to stop lung inflammation and alleviate coughing.
(b) The **_adjuvant_** herbs: "Bai Ji" (*Rhizoma Bletillae*) and "Jie Geng" (*Radix Platycodi*)" to help heal the lung tissue and catalyze the curative effective of the principal herbs.
(c) The **_auxiliary_** herb: "Gan Cao" (*Radix Glycyrrhizae*) to neutralize those possible undesirable effects from the principal and adjuvant herbs.
(d) The **_conductant_** herb: "Ge Gen" (*Radix Puerariae*) to bring the overall curative effect to the Lung meridian; it also brings the heat due to the lung inflammation (i.e. the "rising effect") to the body surface so that it can be dissipated quickly.

In the above discussion, the pneumonia case helps demonstrate how diagnosis and treatment can be achieved by applying the time-honoured axiomatic guidelines and axiomatic principles, which are clearly documented as formalisms in the relevant treatises and Canons. With this information in mind, we can proceed easily to explain the conceptual framework of how herbs are classified in general.

2.4 Herbal Pharmacology

The term herbs in Traditional Chinese Medicine (TCM) should not be taken literally, because, other than plant parts, they also include other material such as minerals, insects, reptiles and animal matter. From the pharmacology TCM viewpoint, herbs can be classified in different ways into different systems according to the set of chosen keys as set out below:

(a) Its association to the Qi channel(s) of the organ(s) as the key: Any herb may associate with one or many Qi channels or organs. For example, "Bai Ji" (*Rhizoma Bletillae*) associates with three organs (and thus three channels), namely, lung, liver, and stomach. Its medicinal effect on each organ may differ; for example, it may be used as a principal herb for the stomach but an adjuvant for the lung. Since the meridians are used as the keys for herbal classifications, Rhizoma Bletillae appears repeatedly in each of the three organs/channels in the final herbal classification system, namely, for the lung, liver and stomach Qi channels or meridians.

(b) Its temperaments as the key: A particular herb may possess one or several of the following properties: heating, cooling, warming, ambient, rising and sinking. For example, "Huang Qin" (*Radix Scutellariae*) is both cooling (i.e. stopping inflammation) and rising (i.e. bringing the heat due to inflammation to the body surface to be dissipated quickly).

(c) Its association with a particular illness: Since a particular herb may be used to treat different illnesses, acting as the principal, adjuvant, auxiliary, or conductant role, we can classify herbs using an illness name or type as the key. This can be achieved by examining the different roles of the same herb when prescribed in previous relevant clinical cases.

If we employ an herbal classification scheme with respect to the set of chosen keywords words (e.g. the 12 Qi channels or organ meridians) a communal ontology [JWong09c], then it is the knowledge base or lexicon by consensus for the community. With this ontology, the communal knowledge can be passed on effectively and unambiguously to the subsequent generations. The standard or consensus-certified vocabulary in the lexicon can be changed only by another new consensus certification in a manual, laborious and communal manner. In TCM there are many communal ontological schemes that exist on top of the knowledge included in the Canons already. The communal ontologies are normally created to suit a particular aim, for example, for industrial standardization, for quick reference of the consultative type, and for enterprise operations. In the case of TCM, communal ontologies are usually subsets extracted from the total/global TCM knowledge embedded in the Canons. A useful industrial/enterprise TCM ontology is well exemplified by PuraPharm's TCM ontological core (or simply onto-core) for computer-aided, web-based clinical practice [JWong09a]. From the proprietary master TCM onto-core, which contains only clinical facts, the PuraPharm Company customizes different computer-aided clinical TCM systems specified by its customers. This is achieved by using a fast-prototyping process called the WD^2UHI (*Web-based Data Mining and Discovery of Useful Herbal Ingredients*) platform [JWong09d]. In Hong Kong many vehicle-based mobile clinics, which are interconnected over the web, are manned by a clinical TCM system customized by PuraPharm (e.g. the famous local YOT (Yan Oi Tong) mobile clinics that treat thousands of patients daily).

2.5 Computer-Aided TCM Takes Various Forms

The TCM domain is wide, and in terms of applications it is associated with our daily lives in the following areas:

(a) Curative: This normally involves the process and treatment by the physician. The physician prescribes the treatment of the diagnosed illness according to the TCM formalisms. The aim is to balance the Yin and Yang [Maciocia05].

(b) Health restoring: In TCM, our food material is also medicine because the food continuum can be divided basically into two categories: curative and dietary.

The curative category usually has potent medicinal properties with specific purposes, for example "Ge Gen" (*Radix Puerariae*) is an efficacious conductant for the lung Qi channel. Yet, it is also a common dietary tuber for making soups for family consumption. When a person is not sick, "Ge Gen" offers dietary advantages: (i) it provides carbohydrates for the body energy, and (ii) it facilitates the body's sweating process to make our body cool in hot weather. In this case "Ge Gen" is health restoring. It is the same for the popular herb "Ren Shen" (*Panax ginseng*), which is the principal herb for many curative prescriptions. But, it is also a common herb for making tea and soup for boosting the body's immune system; it is considered a preventive food material.

Since TCM is associated closely with our daily life and the continuum of food material can be curative and health restoring at the same time, its origin is folk medicine. The transmission of folk medicine at the beginning was from mouth to mouth and from one generation to another. It is customary that a young person in a Chinese village would consult the elders on what to do in order to get well. Therefore, consultation in TCM is not restricted to only the physician but also includes the elders who know the folklore knowledge.

From the above discussion it is clear that computer-aided TCM may take various forms including the following:

(a) Curative: It helps the physician in terms of patients' histories and decision making in the diagnosis/treatment process. A basic curative computer-aided system usually has the following modules: (i) the man/machine interface, (ii) database of patient cases treated by the physician, (iii) accounting (managing the different fees and charges) and (iv) form printing (e.g. prescription forms, and report to the government in case of communicable illnesses)

(b) Consultative: There are different types of consultative systems including the following:

   (i) Type 1—for common/lay use: It lists/explains herbal matters for health restoring, and usually this can be a standalone or supported by different websites that provide the relevant information. If it is web-based, then it is already a form of telemedicine (a minor one) according to the United Nation's definitive concept.

   (ii) Type 2—for common/lay use: It assists anyone to find patent drugs and lists the name of the manufacturers, efficacy statistics, reported side effects and the pharmacies where they can be bought. This type of system is particularly useful for newcomers (e.g. tourists) to a city in emergency cases. Similarly there are also systems that list the medical practitioners, clinics and hospitals in the region so that people can get help. If these systems are web-based, they have already taken the form of telemedicine, however primitive.

   (iii) Type 3—for TCM education: This type of system usually has an architecture of three layers: the first/top layer for the user to input the query; the second/middle layer is the semantic net that interprets/executes the query; the third/bottom layer, which is the database from which the semantic net fetches the required data and returns it to the user as the response to the input query. Again, this type of system can be standalone or web-based.

Within the concept of telemedicine [Lacroix99] the different systems above can be standalone or web-based. In some cases the standalones are interconnected via different networks to achieve the required speed, security, resolution and privacy. In a broad sense, any medical systems that are interconnected via a network indicate their use of telemedicine.

2.6 Contemporary TCM Telemedicine

Contemporary TCM telemedicine is usually ontology-based [Rifaieh06] because the ontological approach allows unambiguous communication and precise answers. It makes use of the idea of the semantic web [W3Ca, W3Cb] so that useful, current scientific TCM discoveries can be data-mined from/via the web. This on-line web mining capability is the backbone of the evolutionary concept of living ontology [JWong08a]. It is reasonable that contemporary TCM Telemedicine should possess at least some of the following characteristics:

(a) Ontology-based: There is always a master ontology from which modular sub-ontologies [JWong09c] can be isolated accurately. In this respect the EOD-ISD type of paradigms may be used.
(b) Global: Since modern telemedicine systems operate on the Internet/web, it is part of a global net knowingly or unknowingly.
(c) Information sharing: The medical practitioner sitting in front of its system (e.g. D/P system) can solicit and import/export information anytime and anywhere around the world.
(d) On-line useful data collection: Using the PuraPharm's pervasive MC-based telemedicine D/P system in Fig. 1.5 as an example, the D/P statistics (e.g. the types of illnesses, the amount of the prescribed herbal ingredients and the likelihood of having communicable illnesses) can be obtained on-line and sent to management and the appropriate authority. With this information the herbs provider management can proactively formulate the ingredients' production plan, and the authority would have more time to plan the preventive measures.
(e) Education: In the past, the medical practitioners had to go to the field to carry out the medical tasks such as diagnosis and prescriptions for treatment in order to get experience. With a telemedicine system such as the PuraPharm D/P system, all the cases treated by different physicians using the same D/P terminal will be stored in a repertoire of personal experiences. This is shown in Fig. 1.8 as the "Experience Window". Normally, only the personal experience of the registered physician who is operating the terminal at the time can be accessed. For educational purposes, all the personal field experience of all the

physicians can be collated into a single file. Then, a trainee can diagnose for the set of artificially input symptoms and then prescribe the corresponding treatment. After that the trainee can compare his/her D/P conclusion with those collated cases in the Experience Window. In the process, the trainee can effectively gain from past experiences gradually.

Living ontology: The information on the web is a treasure trove, and this inspires active research in the area of the semantic web [Taniar06, W3Ca, W3Cb]. Every day there are many new scientific TCM findings reported on the web in various forms and websites. If a telemedicine system can send out data miners to collect these new findings and temporarily append them to the local consensus-certified onto-core in an on-line manner, then several advantages become apparent. The first advantage is that the physician can use these new findings as references in their D/P decisions. The second advantage is that this new and raw data can be part of the information to be considered in the next consensus certification of the update/ migration of the master onto-core [JWong09d].

References

[Lacroix99]   Lacroix, A., Lareng, L., Rossignol, G., Padeken, D., Bracale, M., Ogushi, Y., Wootton, R., Sanders, J., Preost, S., McDonald, I.: G-7 global healthcare applications sub-project 4, international concerted action on collaboration in telemedicine. http://www.atmeda.org/ICOT/finalReport.G8SP.4 (1999). Accessed 10 Jun 2005
[Maciocia05] Maciocia, G.: The Foundations of Chinese Medicine: A Comprehensive Text. Churchill Livingstone, London (2005) (a comprehensive clinical guide)
[Rifaieh06]   Rifaieh, R., Benharkat, A.: From ontology phobia to contextual ontology use in enterprise information system. In: Taniar, D., Rahayu, J. (eds.) Web Semantics and Ontology. Idea Group Incorporated, Hershey (2006)
[Taniar06]   Taniar, D., Rahayu, J. (eds.): Web Semantics and Ontology. Idea Group Incorporated, Hershey (2006)
[JWong08a]   Wong, J.H.K., Dillon, T.S., Wong, A.K.Y., Lin, W.W.K.: Text Mining for Real-time Ontology Evolution, Data Mining for Business Applications, pp. 143–150. Springer, New York (2008). ISBN: 978-0-387-79419-8
[JWong09a]   Wong, J.H.K., Wong, A.K.Y., Lin, W.W.K., Dillon, T.S.: A novel approach to achieve real-time TCM (Traditional Chinese Medicine) telemedicine through the use of ontology and clinical intelligence discovery. Int. J. Comput. Syst. Sci. Eng. (CSSE) **24**, 219–240 (2009)
[JWong09c]   Wong, J.H.K., Lin, W.W.K., Wong, A.K.Y., Dillon, T.S.: TCM (Traditional Chinese Medicine) telemedicine with enterprise ontology support—a form of consensus-certified collective human intelligence. In: Proceedings of the International Conference on Industrial Technology (ICIT), Monash University, Victoria, Australia, 10–13 Feb 2009
[JWong09d]   Wong, J.H.K.: Ph.D. thesis: Web-based Data Mining and Discovery of Useful Herbal Ingredients (**WD²UHI**), Department of Computing, Hong Kong Polytechnic University (2009)
[W3Ca]   W3C: Ontology Definition MetaModel. http://www.omg.org/docs/ad/05-08-01.pdf (2005). Accessed 16 Sept 2005
[W3Cb]   W3C: Web Service Architecture (Working Paper). http://www.w3.org/TR/ws-arch/

Chapter 3
Semantics and Ontology

3.1 Introduction

The web is a worldly information treasure trove, but it contains unorganized knowledge in an intertwined fashion. Usually the meaning and importance of a piece of web information depends on subjective interpretations by the potential users. To benefit a community, subjective interpretations should depend on collective agreements—the prelude to consensus certification.

The *semantic web concept* is an evolving extension of the WWW in which the semantics of information and services on the web are defined. Via some types of interface intelligence, it is possible for the web contents to be understood and to satisfy information retrieval by people and/or machines [Berners01, W3Cc]. It was the vision of Tim Berners-Lee to use the web as a universal medium/platform for data, information and knowledge exchange [Herman08]. In order to achieve this, it is necessary to organize the web with the desired semantics. One way to support this organization is the ontological approach. From the viewpoint of philosophy [Corazzon04], an ontology is a knowledge base that contains consensus-certified items and has a potential evolvable boundary. Usually the concepts, attributes, and the associations among them within the ontology are descriptive, and the formality of the knowledge stems from the process of consensus certification, which constrains interpretation. Yet, it is difficult to force the same constraints for all knowledge domains. One approach to resolving the possible domain-related "multi-representations" for the same items is formulating domain "views", which act like filters/templates to accentuate the desired features and mask out the irrelevant ones. Thus ontology was initially introduced into computing and information technology as a means of providing the semantics in the "Semantic Web". This provided support for the retrieval of information based on its meaning rather than just simple string matching. Since this early use of ontologies, they have grown to provide semantics and mechanisms for communication and structuring of knowledge in a wide variety of uses in IT, Telemedicine, business and many other areas of human

© Springer-Verlag Berlin Heidelberg 2015
A.K.Y. Wong et al., *Semantically Based Clinical TCM Telemedicine Systems*,
Studies in Computational Intelligence 587, DOI 10.1007/978-3-662-46024-5_3

endeavour. In this chapter, we will provide a panoramic vista of some of the ways semantic web and ontologies are being used and that we hope to stimulate more research in the TCM community.

3.2 Ontology

3.2.1 What is an Ontology

Definition Ontology can be viewed as a shared conceptualization of a domain that is commonly agreed to by all parties. It is defined as 'a specification of a Conceptualization' [Gruber93a]. 'Conceptualization' refers to the understanding of the Concepts and relationships between the Concepts that *can* exist or *do* exist in a specific domain or a community. A representation of the shared knowledge in a specific domain that has been commonly agreed to refers to the 'specification' of a Conceptualization.

From this definition, key constructs are 'shared' and 'commonly agreed' knowledge. There is a common misunderstanding about Ontologies. Some people may think *Ontology* is only a set of words, definitions or Concepts, whereas others think Ontology is similar as object-oriented technology or simply a knowledge base.

However, this is not true and these are not Ontologies because the ideas contained in the signifiers 'shared' and 'commonly agreed' must be considered when talking about Ontologies. It is important to note that:

- If some Concepts or knowledge are shared but their meaning is not commonly agreed or vice versa, they are not Ontologies.
- If a set of knowledge is only referred to as Ontology, but nobody uses it and shares it, then they are also not Ontology.
- If a set of Concepts are used to describe objects, they can be shared knowledge within a single application or a single object-oriented system; however, they are not Ontology, because Ontology is for a specific domain not for a specific application.

Ontology is the agreed understanding of the 'being' of knowledge [Hadzic05]. In other words, there is consensus agreement regarding the interpretation of the Concepts and the Conceptual understanding of a domain. Every domain has a commonly used set of Concepts or words, a set of possible closely related meanings to select from. If these Concepts are attributed the same meaning by the community, business parties or domain of service operators, then computers can easily be used to establish communication and carry out tasks automatically. If, within a domain, different parties were to use their own terms and definitions, and there were no translators, then tasks could become very time consuming. It would become virtually impossible for computers to do the tasks automatically using the Internet, especially in the Service Oriented Network or virtual collaborative environment.

A very simple example of an ontological viewpoint of a Concept is a 'Published Article' to include: Author name(s), Article title, Publisher of journal or conference name, or newspaper name, Place published, Date published, and ISBN number, or volume number, or page number. This single Concept can be used cross-culturally and internationally, from the public sector to the private, from groups to individuals.

3.2.2 Generic Ontologies and Specific Ontologies

A domain of interest can be represented by *generic Ontologies* and *specific Ontologies* which are also known as *Upper-Ontology* and *Sub-Ontologies (Lower Ontology)*. The *specific Ontologies* or Sub-Ontologies are also known as *"Ontology commitments"* [Spyns02]. They commit to use all the upper Ontology Concepts and specifications. As an example, a generic concept may be called "human relationship", and a specific "human relationship" concept can be 'boy and girl relationship', or 'business and customer relationship' or 'teacher and student relationship' etc. These are specific relationship concepts and they are all *committed* to the *specification* of the generic concept "human relationship". The *specification* of the generic concept "human relationship" can be defined as "having at least two parties involved. If one party is missing, the relationship would not exist and the Trust Value has no meaning. Therefore, all the Specific Ontologies or Sub-Ontologies should commit to this *specification*.

- Figure 3.1a shows the generic ontological representation of the *Concept* of "Human Relationship";
- Figure 3.1b shows the specific ontological representation of the *Concept* of "Business Relationship"; and
- Figure 3.1c shows the ontological view of Generic and Specific Ontologies or upper and sub-Ontology hierarchy.

The term "Ontology" is derived from its usage in philosophy where it means the study of being or existence as well as the basic categories [Fensel01]. An ontology, in computer science, is an explicit specification of a conceptualisation [Gruber93a,

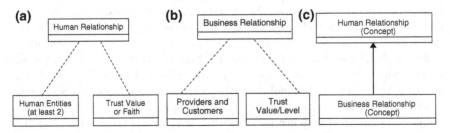

Fig. 3.1 a Ontological representation of generic human relationship concept. **b** Ontological representation of the specific human relationship concept, e.g., business relationship. **c** Generic and specific or upper-sub ontology concept

Gruber93b]. In such an ontology, definitions associate the names of concepts in the universe of discourse e.g. classes, relations, functions with describing what the concepts mean, and formal axioms that constrain the interpretation and well-formed used of these terms [Klein01].

People use the word ontology in different ways and to mean different things. However, different definitions provide different and complementary points of view on the word ontology. In the following sections, we compare ontology with data catalogues of glossaries, data dictionaries, thesauri, taxonomies.

We summarise the comparison between ontology and glossary or data dictionary and a taxonomy form [Dillon93, Noy03]. Ontology is more than a glossary or data dictionary in whose terms everything else must be well described. An Ontology is more than a taxonomy or classification of terms. Often the term 'ontology' has been used very loosely to label almost any conceptual classification schema. Although a taxonomy contributes to the semantics of a term in a vocabulary, ontologies include richer relations between terms. A true ontology should contain not only a hierarchy of concepts organised by 'is a', 'subtype', or 'subclass' relations, but other 'semantic relations' that specify how one concept is related to another. The terms in ontology are chosen to ensure the representation of the abstract foundational concepts and distinctions within the domain of interest and form a complete set whose relationship one to another is defined using formal techniques which provide the semantic basis for the terminology chosen.

We should also distinguish between knowledge representations in Knowledge Based Systems (KBS) and Ontologies. A knowledge representation in a KBS is solely for the purpose of reasoning within that KBS and the terms do not have to be capable of being shared or understood more widely. In contrast, a key element of an ontology is the *shared nature of the conceptualization across the community* which represents the domain.

3.3 The Ontology Argument

The main argument is that the classical ontology can weave/intertwine philosophical knowledge, and this can be achieved by consensus certification—a knowledge engineering approach. Normally, the ontology reflects knowledge up to a particular time t (i.e. $Onto_t$). For example, the philosophical foundations, which were laid down by philosophers such as Aristotle (Greek philosopher) and Lao Zi (Chinese philosopher) have since been expanded as time progresses. It is, however, difficult to realize all the philosophical principles in full. Instead, implementations have to be adapted with respect to the environmental forces, needs, and temporal factors. In the area of computer science, an ontology is considered a viable approach for organizing usable knowledge for scientific and engineering applications. In this light, Gruber [Gruber93a] and Guarino [Guarino00] together have helped lay down a good theoretical basis of how an ontology can be used to disambiguate a "community knowledge base", which should be created by domain experts in a consensus certification process.

The first logical step to reap the potential usefulness of web sources is to organize them into a standard (i.e. community/domain) repertoire. The organization involves: view definitions for terms, attributes, concepts and the associations, classification or categorization of these definitions (sub-ontologies). This is followed by the construction of the corresponding subsumption hierarchy to layout the interconnection among the sub-ontologies. This hierarchy should finally be agreed by consensus to become the "community, domain or enterprise" ontology, which could be made into a machine-usable form. The ontology approach makes the web semantics potentially usable, and from the user's point of view, the web is now semantic (i.e. meanings can be easily extracted and used—semantic web). If one could transform the subsumption hierarchy in the web ontology into a Petri net, then every network/ semantic/operation path (in the Petri net) would have a meaning (semantic). Then, tracing such a path for a set of parameters is a logical process or inference. The final path traced out by the inference process is the logical conclusion for the given set of parameters. The connotation of every distinctive semantic path can be predefined in the specific context via a consensus certification process.

The concept of problem domains and the application of specific salient features arouse the concept of portable ontology specifications. Gruber proposed that any computer-application ontology should have the following high-level characteristics [Gruber93a]:

(a)   It is an *explicit specification of a conceptualization* that caters to: (i) representation of the consensus-certified domain knowledge (e.g. human disease [Wongthongtham06b] and allopathic medicine [UMLS]); (ii) the ontology should have a logical representation or machine-understandable form (i.e. the semantic net that is alternatively known as the DOM (document object model) in the W3C area); and (iii) the corresponding human-understandable form (i.e. the syntactical layer for implicit or explicit query formations). Therefore, a system with ontology support should have three layers: ontology at the bottom, a semantic net (and the corresponding parsing mechanism or parser) in the middle, and a query system at the top. The parser provides the logical conclusion for the query according to its actual parameters specified by the user by working at the DOM tree by inference.

(b)   The knowledge in the form of descriptive philosophy must be translated correctly into the application knowledge/data.

The second characteristic in Gruber's proposal is not easy to achieve as it involves the issue of appropriate and flexible data structures as well as the issue of supporting interoperability. Today, the computer is basically the web or Internet even within a commercial enterprise. Sharing the same ontological knowledge/data base over the web may involve machines, communication technologies, and software from various vendors [Hamilton02]. In order to confine the meaning of Gruber's second characteristics in the field of applications, Guarino proposed that the ontological contents should be organized into a subsumption hierarchy [Guarino00], and the interpretation of the associations among sub-ontologies should be axiomatically constrained. This proposal had alleviated the ontology phobia of many potential applicants [Taniar06]. Since then, building an enterprise ontology to house the necessary knowledge of an enterprise or corporation has started to flourish [Clark05, Coplien04, Dunn05, JWong09b, JWong09d]. There was obvious success in adopting the enterprise concept for managing software development, which involves different teams across the globe (i.e. *multi-site software development*). If the ontology is the enterprise vocabulary with constrained interpretation that all the team involved must use it as a base, then there is no chance for multi-representation of the same terms; modules can be integrated seamlessly [JWong08b].

Meanwhile, different groups have been actively researching how to support the translation process (Gruber's 2nd characteristic), and it has been generally concluded that the use of metadata (e.g. XML, RDF, and OWL) is a viable approach [Lopez99, IBM03]. Other researchers have been busy proposing ontology building and managing tools [Denny04], but unfortunately these tools are often exclusively inoperable. One conclusion, however, is seemingly unanimous—we can use semantic web technology to integrate enterprises—and the W3C has contributed tremendously in this aspect. Indirectly, the accumulated XML, RDF, and OWL metadata experience in the field has benefited this research direction enormously.

In fact, the ultimate aim of using ontology is to disambiguate information interchange by constraining terminology with respect to the standard community vocabulary/lexicon. If the "community knowledge base" is for usage within an enterprise, it would be the enterprise knowledge base or enterprise ontology. The constraining process disallows certain meanings of the same word (i.e. multi-representations). To put this into perspective, the meanings of terms are filtered so that only those relevant meanings are allowed to pass through; these filters are the domain/application views. A successful example is an enterprise ontology for "distributed software engineering", which may involve different groups in different regions/countries across the globe (e.g. Verizon). The enterprise ontology supported by predefined views filters out regional multi-representations for the same term, making software modules developed anywhere, anytime "integrate-able" with minimal errors. A key ontology feature is that, through formal, real-world semantics and consensual terminologies, it interweaves human and machine understanding [Fensel03]. In this way, the ontology facilitates sharing and reuse of knowledge for both humans and machines.

The UMLS [UMLS] is a real-life example of how the concept of ontology is realized successfully in the area of Western/allopathic medicine. The UMLS is organized into three layers: (i) the allopathic context, from a specific angle, into the bottom-layer ontology; (ii) the middle-layer semantic net to logically represent the bottom ontology for machine processing; it is the machine process-able form and the processor is the logical parser; and (iii) the top-layer syntactical representation of the semantic net so that human users can formulate the corresponding queries. In fact, all three layers connote the same knowledge in different forms for different purposes. The knowledge, however, must be represented formally and in a retrievable form for practical use. The representation or retrieval form can be a metadata system (e.g. XML). For production systems the meta-system may be converted into technology-oriented databases (e.g. Microsoft (MS) relational database—SQL server) so that tools from different vendors are readily applicable.

In this way the chance of premature obsolescence is prevented because the databases are tied in with the related proprietary artefacts of data interoperability. This also applies to the metadata systems; for example, XML, RDF and OWL have less chance of obsolescence because they are supported by the influential W3C and many vendors (e.g. IBM and Microsoft).

As the semantic web keeps developing [Fensel03], its knowledge content is becoming richer and more useful. As a result it should be managed to the benefit of mankind on a global scale. Tim Berners-Lee actually envisioned the semantic web as the natural evolution from the current web. Its evolution involves additions of machine-readable information and automated services. Berners-Lee thought that explicit representations of semantics underlying the web data, programs, pages, and other web resources would support qualitative new services [Fensel03].

3.4 Ontology Modelling Notation

In this section, we present a notation system for *Ontology Representation*. This is because in the literature so far, there is no standard for Ontology Representation. A well-known notation such as UML, UML2 has limited power to represent the Ontology and causes confusion between Object Technology and Ontologies. OWL contains a powerful representation of Ontologies. However, it is not readily understandable by domain experts. Hence, we define a notation system for an Ontology using a graphical representation. We have chosen simplicity for ease of understanding and give a clear semantic for each of the constructs used.

There are 5 key notations or constructs, namely:

- Ontology Concept/Ontology Classes
- Ontology Instance
- Ontology Association Relation
- Ontology Generic-Specific Relation
- Ontology Include/Part-of Relation

Notation 1—Ontology Concept
An Ontology Concept is defined as an abstraction of agreed terms, definitions and vocabularies. A Concept is an important element in modelling and representing reality. A Concept is an abstraction that captures the properties of a group of individual instances that have commonalities. The Concept is defined by its intention or extension. The intension of a Concept is a specification that gives a definition of its properties and the axioms related to it. This gives a definition of its structure and behaviours. The extension of the Concept is the enumeration of all its instances and relations.

In many proposed Ontology Modelling Languages, the notion of Concept is used interchangeably with the notion of Class. However, in Ontology modelling, it is important to recognise that a Concept has to be shared across the domain and is

Table 3.1 Notation for representing ontology concept

Ontology notation	Semantics of the notation
	Double-field box represents the *ontological concept*

Note:
• Each concept has its own specification, including hierarchical or association relations with other concepts, attributes, etc. In this chapter, many examples are given

• "Specification of the concept" means specify the common agreed definitions or axioms which are satisfied by every ontology instance of the concepts. This is the intension of the concept. It can also be specified by enumerating the instances of the concept or extension of the concept

commonly agreed between the participants in the domain. This is in contrast to the case of class/object in Object-Oriented Modelling or Knowledge Modelling in Knowledge Based Systems where the system modeller dictates the definition of the class/object.

Concept can be organized in generalisation/specialisation hierarchies, or part of hierarchies and have association relationships with other Concepts (Table 3.1).

Notation 2—Ontology Instance
An Ontology Instance is defined as a specific individual Ontology Concept or example of the Concept (Table 3.2).

Table 3.2 Notation for representing ontology instance

Ontology notation	Semantics of the notation
	Circle-line represents the instance of ontological concept

Note:
• In Ontology, it does not matter whether it is in the upper or sub class concepts, as they can all have "instances"

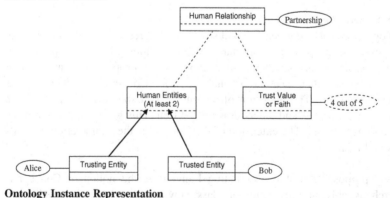

Ontology Instance Representation

Notation 3—Ontology Association Relation
Association Relation is defined as *a relation which represents one Concept is closely related to another Concept or Concepts. It expresses a dependency between Concepts.* The association relation is sometimes annotated with a name giving it specific semantics (Table 3.3).

Notation 4—Generic and Specific Ontology Relation
Generic-Specific Ontology Relation expresses the generalisation/specialisation relation between the upper Ontology Concept which is a generalization and a Sub-Ontology Concept which is a specialisation. The Sub or Lower Ontology Concept or Concepts must commit to all the specifications of the Upper Ontology Concept. The specific Ontology involves additional constraints which specify the specialisation (Table 3.4).

Notation 5—Composition/Part-of Ontology Relation
The Ontology Composition/Part-of relation is defined as *a composition of lower level Concepts to form an upper level composite* Concept. The lower level Concepts are in a 'part of' relation to the upper level Concept (Table 3.5).

Table 3.3 Notation for representing ontology association relation

Ontology notation	Semantics of the notation
- - - - - - - - - - - - - - - - -	A dotted line represents the ontology association relation, which represents that a concept is closely related to another concept. The cardinality and characteristics of the concept association can be added on the top of the dotted line

Note:
• The association relation between the concepts is an important part of the ontology representation. Often, one concept is related to another concept. It is important to comprehend this and the concepts themselves to understand its full semantics within a context

• Here, the focus is concept "dependency" rather than "relationship" between the concepts. Therefore, the cardinality is not central. However, for implementation constraints, if necessary, the notation "1:0, 1:1, 1:M or M:M" to express cardinality can be added

• Here, the association relationship can be further classified by its relationship characteristics, such as one of the following:
- Explicit association
- Implicit association
- Asymmetry
- Transitivity
- Antonymy (or Inverse)
- Asynchrony
- Gravity

The notation to express the characteristics of the relationship is to add ≪ Character ≫ on the top of the dotted line. Such as

Explicit — — — — — — — Transitive — — — — — — — Asymmetry — — — — etc

In OWL, four association relationships is distinguished, they are named as "Functional", "Symmetric", "Transitive" and "Inverse"

Table 3.4 Notation for representing generic-specific ontology relation

Ontology notation	Semantics of the notation
⟶	Line with solid arrow represents *the generalisation and specialisation relation*, which is a relation between upper-lower *generic and specific* concepts

Note:
• The generalisation and specialisation relation is defined as *the relation between a super-class Concept and a sub-class concept.* The sub-class concept inherits the properties of the super-class concept

Table 3.5 Notation for representing include/part-of ontology relation

Ontology notation	Semantics of the notation
⟹	Line with open arrow represents composition and aggregation or part-of relationship between upper ontology concept and lower ontology concept

Note:
• In an ontology presentation, we can distinguish part-of relation from *generalisation and specialisation* hierarchical relation and part-of relationship is a kind of aggregation relationship that may be mutually inclusive, exclusive or only part-of

• The upper ontology concept may be a composite with a number of parts, and the lower ontology concepts are 'part of' the upper ontology concept

• The composition/part-of relations can form a hierarchy

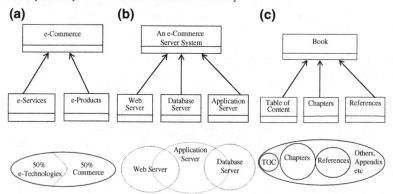

(a) Exclusive Aggregation
(b) Inclusive Aggregation
(c) Partial include or Part of

• In Ontology, once a concept hierarchy is created, there is a consideration of whether it is making sense from the reverse point of view. For example, if a hierarchy is built from left to right, the reverse view is from right to left. In object/class relationships, the reverse view is very important and it always must be the case

Table 3.6 Ontology notation summary

Ontology notation	Semantics of the notation
(double-field box)	Double-field box represents the *ontological concept*
(circle-line)	Circle-line represents the instance of ontological concept
- - - - - - - - - - - - - - -	A dotted line represents ontology concept association relation which represents a concept is closely related to another concept
⟶ (solid arrow)	Line with solid arrow represents *the generalisation and specialisation relation*, which is a relation between upper-lower *generic and specific* concepts
⟹ (open arrow)	Line with open arrow represents composition and aggregation or part-of relationship between upper ontology concept and lower ontology concept

A more complete presentation is given in Appendix 1

Summary of Ontology Notation

In this section, we give a summary of five most important notations that are frequently used in Ontology Representations (Table 3.6).

3.5 Purposes for Which Ontologies are Being Used

Ontologies are being used in our research for several purposes. These include:

1. To provide a strong and unambiguous communication mechanism, and references medium for TCM Practitioners working at multiple sites to develop solutions to a problem they are dealing with, the TCM ontology has a critical role to play.
2. To provide a mediating mechanism for accessing heterogeneous data and information sources, particularly on the Web.
3. To enable the building of applications on the Web by providing clearly defined semantics for Web services.
4. To provide a common knowledge base for multi agents working in a particular domain.
5. To provide clearly defined semantics and confidence for interactions on the Web, more specifically, to build:

   (a)   Trust and Reputation systems [Chang06]
   (b)   Privacy Based systems [Hecker08, Hecker06]

6. To provide clearly defined semantics for the knowledge in a number of different domains, including:

- disease ontology
- treatment ontology
- manufacturing ontology
- different financial systems ontologies

It will not be possible in the space of this chapter to discuss each of these ontologies in detail and their use. We will therefore make a selection and discuss some cases.

3.5.1 Strong and Unambiguous Communication Mechanism

There are four issues that need to be addressed:

- Communication and coordination
- Unified Knowledge Sharing
- Knowledge Sharing Platform
- Methodology Adaptation and Validation

Failure to identify a clear issue or to correctly interpret an answer, often causes miscommunication, misunderstanding, and misinterpretations during discussion, subsequently followed by the lack of coordination of activities and tasks. The physical distance becomes a crucial issue when the specifications are not complete, or ambiguous, or continually evolving, thereby needing more interaction among team members. Failure to share unifying knowledge, which includes domain knowledge, common knowledge, and project information including project data, project agreement, and project understanding, is a key issue. Awareness of the work that is being done according to the plan, the work that is being done co-operatively between teams, the current issues that have been raised, the issues that have been clarified, and the means whereby members can conduct a discussion in order to make a decision on issues, all present a challenge in a multi-site distributed environment. Different teams might not be aware of the tasks that are being carried out by others, potentially leading to problems such as two groups overlapping in some work, or other work not being performed due to misinterpretation of the task. Wrong tasks may be carried out due to ignorance of whom to contact in order to obtain the proper details. If everyone working on a certain project being located in the same area, then situational awareness is relatively straightforward. Over the last three years, we have developed the world's first and only Software Engineering Ontology (SE Ontology) which is available online at www.seontology.org. The SE Ontology defines common sharable software engineering knowledge including particular project information [Wongthongtham06a, Wongthongtham06b] and typically provides software engineering concepts—what the concepts are, how they are related, and why they are related [Wongthongtham06a, Wongthongtham06b]. These concepts facilitate common understanding of software engineering project information to all the distributed members of a development team in a multi-site development environment. We have merged Gruber's [Gruber93a, Gruber93b], and Studer's [Studer98] definitions of an ontology as a basis to define the software engineering ontology. Hence, the software engineering ontology is a formal, explicit specification of a shared conceptualisation in the domain of software engineering. 'Formal' implies that the software engineering ontology should be machine-understandable. Software engineering ontology facilitates better communication over software engineering domain knowledge between humans and machines. 'Explicit' implies that the type of software engineering concepts used, and their constraints, are explicitly defined. Software engineering ontology standardises and formalises the meaning of terms in the software engineering through its concepts. 'Shared' shows that the ontology specifies consensual knowledge of software engineering which means it is public and accepted by a group of software engineers. 'Conceptualisation' implies an abstract model that has identified the relevant software engineering concepts.

It is not necessary that an ontology has instances, but the TCM ontology has the instances that represent project information including project data, project understanding, and project agreement.

3.5.2 Ontology Mediated Information Access

In any given field of databases, there are widely varying characteristics using their own categories for storing data. Sometimes, different databases use identical labels but with different meanings; conversely, the same meanings are expressed via different names. Whenever database interoperability becomes a major problem, an ontology has a major role to play in alleviating this situation. For example, in one database whose entity relationship diagram is shown in Fig. 3.2, data about an activity transition (transition between activities) might be encoded for the activity transition together with branch transition (transition between activities through the condition), special transition (transition from an activity to a stop or transition from

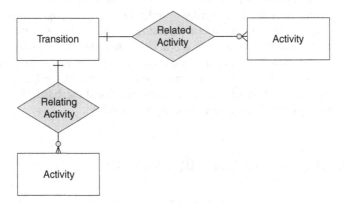

Fig. 3.2 Entity relationship diagram representing activity transition concept

a start to an activity) and concurrent transition (transition between activities through either a fork or a join). In the ontology, these transitions are separated; therefore queries about fork transition, for instance, can be directed to the right place.

Rules in ontology can be expressed about relationships between concepts or classes and these can be used in query processing that generates all results matching the query according to the specified relationships. Unlike databases, in an ontology, new facts can be generated by inferring or reasoning with the asserted facts.

There has been a Data Explosion of Protein Structure Data which makes it difficult to create explanatory and predictive models that are consistent with the huge volume of data. This difficulty increases when a large variety of heterogeneous approaches to gather data from multiple perspectives and store it with completely different formats in the different protein databases. In order to facilitate computational processing of the data from the multiple data sources, we have built the first and only available Protein Ontology (PO) to integrate protein knowledge and provide a structured and unified vocabulary to represent protein synthesis concepts [Sidhu06]. This PO:

- consists of concepts, which are data descriptors for proteomics data and the relationships among these concepts.
- has:
  - a hierarchical classification of concepts represented as classes, from general to specific.
  - a list of attributes related to each concept, for each class.
  - a set of relationships between classes to link concepts in ontology in more complicated ways then implied by the hierarchy, to promote reuse of concepts in the ontology.
  - a set of algebraic operators for querying protein ontology instances.

More details about Protein Ontology are at: http://www.proteinontology.info. The Protein Ontology is a part of Standardized Biomedical Ontologies available through the National Center for Biomedical Ontologies along with Gene Ontology, Flybase, and others. http://cbioapprd.stanford.edu/ncbo/faces/pages/ontology_list. xhtml. This PO will form a standard on accessing the different protein data sources.

As the ontology in this application can act as a mediator for accessing not only relational data but also semi-structured data such as XML or metadata annotations and unstructured information it is a generalization of the original concept of a mediator proposed by Weiderhold for accessing relational databases. We call this approach Ontology Mediated Information Access (OMIA).

3.5.3   Ontology and Semantic Web Services

Web services [Alonso04, Shadbolt06, Chang06] are self-contained components applications that can be described, published, located, and invoked over internet.

Web Services can be dynamically composed into applications. And this allows the implementations to be platform independent and programming language-neutral. Web Services systems promote significant decoupling and dynamic binding of components. The independence of different services publishers and the subscribers can formulate the most suited services they want.

Software as a service is going to be increasingly the dominant means of delivery and consumption of software. This will mean there must be a good enough characterization of the semantics of the services to allow one to choose the appropriate service and to compose different components of software that meet particular requirements. In addition, this will introduce new approaches to software development. TCM Practitioners are often working at multi sites and hence we need to allow one to cost-effectively access the resources to carry out the diagnosis and treatment. This brings new challenges in communication between the TCM practitioners working at different sites. Here again, ontologies have an important role to play.

The contemporary web services specification models merely focus on the *syntactical* levels, e.g. the Web Service Definition Language (WSDL), the Web Services Flow Language (WSFL), the Business Process Execution Language for Web Services (BPEL4WS), Web Service Capability Description Language (SCDL). Web Service Choreography Service (WSCI). These schemes capture the structural properties of the web components only, using the BPEL and WSCI to weave different Web services into meaningful business processes. However, this still remains a specification at the syntactic level. It is likely that the requirements of a user will often not be met by a single web service but will require the composition of several component web services.

There are several issues that must be addressed for successful application of these web services and these include: (1) selection of a suitable architecture—see [Dillon07a, Dillon07b] for a discussion of different architectural styles and a proposed new approach; (2) Discovery of suitable services [Wu07]; (3) selection of a service; and (4) composition and coordination of the services to meet the requirements. To assist the process particularly of discovery and selection our group like several other researchers have decided that it is necessary to semantically annotate these web services. We use a combination of Ontologies and Web 2.0 philosophy to achieve provision of semantics and composition. The key ideas below are more fully explained in [Dillon07a, Dillon07b].

First we define a core concept: a **Service Space** is a supportive environment where a collection of Web services gather for the purpose of fulfilling user demands. Service space is the 'first class' concept to cope with challenges inherent in distributed Web services. It should be noted that a service space does not host, manage, or run services as do most services containers [Dhesiaseelan04]. Rather, it provides infrastructure to enable service discovery and "mashup" at various levels. Web services within a Service Space are referred to as 'members' of that Service Space. In the Service Space regular Web resources are 'augmented' to Semantic Web Services which are then integrated into various Virtual Organisations in response to user requirements from the application layer. Three major Service Spaces are defined for 'lifting up' Web services, i.e. the Web Service Space, the Semantic Web Space, and the Virtual Organisation Space. In While Web 2.0 technology and 'attitude' [Lin06] are to be entrenched in all three types of service spaces, they are particularly helpful in building Semantic Web Space and Web Service Space respectively.

The **Web Service space** provides fundamental infrastructure that enables the discovery of a large number of basic Web services in a loosely-coupled manner regardless of their locations, categories, and qualities. From the perspective of the Service-Oriented Computing, it resembles a number of contemporary global Web service registries such as public UDDI Business Registry, XMethods, StrikeIron, IBM SOA Catalog, etc. that can facilitate essential keyword-based service discovery. It also supports service subscription that allows potential *users* to track down interesting Web services.

Semantic Web Space (SWS) refers to a focused *Service Space* where a group of related Web services forms a domain-specific Web service community in order to facilitate dependable collaboration through trust-driven service selection and semantic-based service discovery. Domain here refers to areas with limited boundaries such as a specific geographical region, a particular industry, etc. Semantic Web Space shall provide sufficient elements for the establishment and enforcement of trust for users [Chang06] and 'sense of community' for member Web services. We have recently observed that numerous Web 2.0 communities (e.g. 43things, Youtube, MySpace, del.icio.us) prosper for various reasons that can be studied in a number of disciplines including economy, social science, biology, and information science. The Semantic Web Space respects this phenomenon. Moreover, it utilises and extends such 'collective intelligence' by providing formal semantic-enabled and semantic-aware instruments that help to build long-lasting Web service communities are beneficial for all Web service providers and consumers.

Transient Virtual Organisation (VO) is a demand-driven *Service Space* that allows a small group of Web services to form an ad hoc team working collectively in order to fulfil particular user demands during a given period of time. The main reasons for spawning such a transient VO lies in the gap between the complexity of actual user requirements and the limitation of each individual Web service obtained from both Web Service Space and Semantic Web Space. In addition, we believe ad hoc **Web service mashup**—Web service mediation, expansion, customisation, and integration are essential for a VO to satisfy real-world user requirements. Presumably, VO members often come from the same Semantic Web Space so that most collaboration grounding—trust establishment, shared mission and value, agreed-upon business protocol, and essential technical interfaces, etc.—has been addressed by the semantic-based augmentation prior to the SWS formation. This well-established SWS is defined as the **enclosing SWS** of the VO. During the VO member selection, preferences are given to enclosing SWS members. It is however possible that external Web services are sometimes 'invited' to join a VO in case that appropriate Web services cannot be found solely from a single *enclosing SWS*. It is also possible that a SWS member is engaged in several VOs. In this case, the proportion of its commitment to a particular VO becomes an important criterion for the VO member selection. A group of End Users or a Broker conducts in-depth search in the Web Service Space and selectively collects Web services from various providers into several Semantic Web Spaces based on interests and the semantics of these Web services. During this process, a great number of anarchic Web services are 'clustered' into a well-organised Semantic Web Space dedicated in one specific domain. In general, we envisage that one can apply two approaches to semantically enrich existing Web services. The first top-down approach is based on the concept of ontology engineering, where scientists and domain experts manually annotate relevant Web services using specific domain ontologies and/or knowledge databases. The second empirical approach builds on practical methods such as data/text mining, business intelligence, machine learning that can be carried out (semi-) automatically without intensive human involvement. The Semantic Web Space nurtures Web services mainly through three means: semantic enrichment, semantic classification, and semantic discovery. A Broker directly deals with End User's demands and selects appropriate Web services from existing Semantic Web Space to conduct **Web Service Mashup**—a process where related Web services are rapidly integrated, customised, expanded, and mediated in an ad hoc manner – in order to form a Virtual Organisation fulfilling the customer requirements. Our previous work in [Chang06] has made the first endeavours to address service assessment and selection using the trust model and methodology. Instead of relying exclusively on the Service Broker, end users can also track down constantly-changing Web services in any Service Spaces through the user-centred **Web Service Portal** (WSP). A WSP refers to a locally-accessible and highly-customisable user interface that provides a personalised view of activities and information essential to performing Service Space functions. In other words, WSP acts as a proxy on behalf of the end users to maintain a list of communication channels to involved Service Spaces. Unlike a traditional HTTP proxy server shared by a group of corporate users, a WSP is dedicated to serve only one user, thus creating the 'user-centred' view. WSP also reveals the notion of 'User Mashup'—a core concept underpinning the attitude of Web 2.0 [Högg06]. **User Mashup** in the context of WSP refers to an activity in which the user can 'hack' standard Service Space communication protocols, and hence extensively customises user interface or features based on his own preferences. User Mashup has a far-reaching influence on the development of the user-centred Service Space. It endows users with a broader control over the information flow across the Service Space as well as a refined user experience seamlessly integrated with end user applications in a loosely-coupled manner. Most significantly, User Mashup provides a powerful yet simple mechanism by which infinite 'virtual' syndications of Service Spaces can be created for each WSP. A **Virtual Syndication** of Service Spaces is a fresh, highly filtered, and combinatory view of several Services Spaces within a WSP. It is created, customised, and solely owned by each individual SSP user and does not affect other users or existing Service Spaces in any ways.

These ideas have also been extended to semantic Grid Services in [Dillon07b].

3.5.4 Ontology Based Multi Agent Systems

Agents are software entities capable of autonomous action. To solve more complex problems, a collection of agents that collaborate to solve problems in a given domain are employed and these systems are referred to as Multi Agent Systems. Frequently these agents have a small knowledge base to endow them with some intelligence. The problem always remains of ensuring that the knowledge bases of the different agents are coherent and consistent with one another. One solution to this is to have an ontology which is shared by all the agents in a given domain. The collection of agents in the Multi Agent System could then utilise this ontology as their common knowledge base. This will considerably facilitate communication and coordination between the agents when they are collaborating to solve a problem. However one of the problems that has remained until recently is that while there are methodologies for developing an ontology and methodologies for developing Multi Agent systems they are quite separate and do not have any link or connection with one another. As the key aspect is putting the Multi Agent System and Ontology together to leverage of each other, it is important that the methodology for developing one takes account of the other. This issue has led to the group at DEBII developing a Methodology for Integrated Multi Agent and Ontology Development and the research is reported in [Hadzic08].

3.6 Ontology Modelling and Representation

When developing an ontology model or representation one should be cognizant of:

- Generic ontologies (upper ontologies) and specific ontologies (sub-ontologies, lower ontologies).
- Specific ontologies commit to use all the upper ontology concepts and specifications.

    …

E.g. 'human relationship' is a generic concept while 'boy and girl relationship' or 'business and customer relationship' or 'teacher and student relationship' are specific forms of this generic concept.

To represent an ontology, processes should include a set of tasks as following:

- Define **concepts and concept hierarchy in generic ontology** e.g. define human relationship concept.
- Define **ad hoc relationships** e.g. define relationship of human entities.
- Define **constraints of each relationship** e.g. define as having at least two entities involved.
- Define **concepts and concept hierarchy in specific ontology** e.g. define business relationship concept specific to human relationship concept.

Define **instances of ontological concepts in the specific ontology** e.g. Alice can be defined as one of the human entities having a relationship with another human entity i.e. Bob. Alice and Bob are both instances of human entities.

When modelling Ontologies, we need to be aware of various formalisms for modelling ontologies such as Knowledge Interchange Format (KIF) and knowledge representation languages descended from KL-ONE. KIF has a Lisp-like syntax to express sentences of first order predicate logic. Descendants of KL-ONE use description logics or terminological logics that provide a formal characterisation of the representation.

Those representations have had little success outside Artificial Intelligent (AI) research laboratories. AI knowledge representation has a linear syntax but no standard graphical representation. We have borrowed some **UML-like Figures** to define the abstract syntax, semantics, and notations as an alternative formalism. UML has difficulty modelling ontologies.

The notations further structure into **metamodels/diagrams** which are logically structured.

- Make it simple and easy to understand.
- Enable it to capture the semantic richness of the defined ontology modelling.
- Use a Semi-formal graphical representation for specifying and modelling the ontology.

We need to take care of:

- **Ontology instances** represent concrete information specified as an instance of one or several **ontology classes**. Links between ontology instances represent their interactions.
- **Ontology properties** represent binary relationships held among ontology classes/ontology instances.
- **Ontology classes**

   Ontology classes are organised into a superclass-subclass hierarchy.
   Ontology classes:

- An ontology class can be a superclass of more than one ontology class allow for **multiple inheritance**.
- An ontology class can take the form of **complex descriptions**. The complex descriptions can be built up using simpler ontology class descriptions that are bound together using logical operation i.e. OR (U) and AND (∩).

   - A union ontology class is created by combining two or more ontology classes using the OR operator (U).
   - An intersection ontology class is created by intersecting two or more ontology classes using the AND operator (∩).

- Two **conditions** to describe an ontology class: "necessary condition" and "necessary and sufficient condition"

Ontology properties:

- can have inverses.
- can be limited to having a single value.
- can be transitive or symmetric.
- are used to create restrictions to restrict the ontology instances that belong to an ontology class.
- are also known as roles in Description Logic, are roughly equivalent to relationships in the usual conceptual model used in software engineering and are quite close to attributes in object-oriented modelling.

We model the ontology with generalisation, partition (or aggregation), decomposition, disjoint, and association relationships. If we implement the ontology in OWL, the part-of relationship is implemented as partition.

3.7   Differentiating Conceptual Modelling for Data Modelling, Knowledge Modelling and Ontology Modelling and a Notation for Ontology Modelling

- There has been considerable debate over the relationship between conceptual models for:
  - data modelling
  - knowledge modelling
  - ontology modelling
- Suitable notations for representation of the ontology models:
  - Considerable work has been done on representations for.
  - Implementation of ontologies.
  - Formal semantics based on description logics.

Less work has been directed towards a representation that is in a form suitable for domain experts and non-computer scientists to understand and critique an ontology model. This is necessary as domain experts can pick up inaccuracies, inconsistencies and incompleteness in a proposed ontology. This has previously been found to be very useful for data modelling, software modelling and knowledge modelling [Dillon93]. In this chapter we will address these issues.

Ontology Definition

Before discussing the above issues, it is useful to briefly review the ontology definitions again. Amongst the definitions and descriptions of ontologies we note the following:

- An Ontology is a **shared** conceptualization of a domain that is **commonly agreed** to by all parties, 'a specification of a conceptualization' [Gruber93a].

- An Ontology means to facilitate knowledge reuse by different applications, software systems and human resources. Ontologies are highly expressive knowledge models and they increase **expressiveness and intelligence** of a system.

There are frequent misunderstandings of an ontology and these include, for example: an ontology is only a set of words, definitions or concepts; ontology is similar to an object-oriented model; and an ontology is simply a knowledge base. Note that:

- If some concepts or knowledge is shared but the **meaning is not commonly agreed** or vice versa, they are not ontologies.
- If a set of knowledge is only referred to as ontology, **but nobody uses it or shares it**, then it is also not ontology.
- If a set of concepts is used to describe objects, it can be shared knowledge within a single application or a single object-oriented system; however, it is not ontology, because an ontology is for a specific domain and **not for a specific application**.

We next examine the difference between Ontology Modelling and Design Versus Data Modelling [Dillon08, Guarino00, Hadzic08]. Ontologies and data models both represent domain knowledge but there are some fundamental differences.

Useful points of reference when making the comparison are [Spyns02]:

- Application dependencies
- Knowledge coverage
- Expressive power
- Operation levels

In considering application dependencies, one can note that:

- Data models are designed to fulfil specific needs and therefore depend on the **specific tasks** that need to be performed. **Users, goals, purposes and intended use of the model** influence the modelling process and the level of detail described by this model. Application requirements for the limited set of applications are likely to use the data base, therefore, of considerable importance in defining the data model. Also terms used in the data model to describe entities in the data model frequently use acronyms as they are meant to be largely used by the system developers.
- In contrast, ontologies are **generic and task-independent as possible**. A **minimum of application requirements** are considered during the ontology design. The Ontology consists of relatively **generic knowledge that can be reused by different kinds of applications across a community of users**.

If the application does not require specific knowledge, the data model will be designed without it, as relevance to the applications is of primary importance in specifying the data model.

In contrast, ontologies represent agreed and shared knowledge for the domain. So, the fact that some knowledge describes an aspect of a domain means that it must be represented in the ontology even though no target applications maybe apparent that are going to use this knowledge.

When considering knowledge coverage we note that:

- Data models focus on establishing correspondence between **organization of the data in databases** and **concepts for which the data is being stored**.
- In contrast, ontologies are concerned with the **understanding of the knowledge by community members**. Ontologies are more complete representation of concepts and relationships.

Ontologies have more expressive power compared to the data models; ontology languages are more expressive languages as they include constructs that express other kinds of meaningful constraints such as taxonomy or inferencing. Ontology languages make the domain conceptualization more correct and precise. **Ontologies** are generic, task and implementation-independent and as such operate on a **higher level of abstraction**. In contrast, **data models** are at the **lower level of abstraction**.

In considering operation levels we consider the following illustrative example from the Car domain [Dillon08, Guarino00, Hadzic08]:

- a **'new car database'** would model a car using attributes such as model and make of car, pricing, colour, engine size, accessories; a **'repair database'** might model spare parts associated with a particular model and make of a car, their price, the price for the labour to fit in the spare part, result ranges for certain tests, etc. Both of these data models have a narrow view of the concepts of a car suitable to the application.
- **A Car Ontology** can be designed to represent the knowledge common and shared by both 'new car database' and 'repair database'. This knowledge will operate on a higher level of abstraction and will be designed independently from the applications running on each of these databases.

Next we examine the difference between an Ontology Versus a Knowledge Base. Ontologies and Knowledge bases both represent domain knowledge, but there are some fundamental differences and these include the following:

- An ontology **captures and represents the conceptual structure of a domain** in a form that is **shared by the community of users** in that domain.
- In contrast, a knowledge base models knowledge in that domain in a form suitable for a particular Knowledge-Based System (KBS) to **carry out problem solving**. Knowledge base models the problem solver's (expert's) approach to problem solving for the particular set of problems being addressed within this domain. Knowledge base enables an inference engine or agent to reason to solve the particular set of problems that the KBS is meant to address.
- An ontology has **terminology and conceptualization agreed on by the community to be correct and to be consistently used across the community**.

- Whilst in the KBS, the **terminology can be specific to the particular system** and consistency is understood to mean logical consistency within the narrow focus of the problems being solved.
- The purpose of an ontology is to describe **facts assumed to be always true by the community of users**. It aims to capture the conceptual structures of a domain.
- In contrast, the knowledge base aims to **specify the portion of the domain useful for solving a particular set of problems**. It may also describe facts related to a particular state of affairs.
- For an agent, a shared ontology describes a **vocabulary for communicating about a domain**.
- In contrast, a knowledge base contains the **knowledge needed to solve problems or answer queries about such a domain**. **Domain knowledge** is described by ontologies while **operational knowledge** is described in the knowledge base.

These differences between an ontology and a knowledge base are summarised in Table 3.7.

The above discussion of the connection between Ontologies and Databases leads to an understanding of how Ontologies can support data models. Thus:

- **Ontologies** can be used to **build, support and clarify data models**.
- An ontology can play an important role during the data model design, especially in the requirements analysis.

A wide range of ontologies is available via **ontological libraries** and these can be used to assist in the modelling of a specific application domain. Also, **data models** may **support the ontology design process in the following way**:

- Data models may help to provide knowledge that will help designers make decisions regarding **organization and structuring of the concepts within an ontology** [Zhao08]. This is particularly the case if we trace entities back to the user interface for the database.

Table 3.7 Differences between an ontology and a knowledge base

	Ontology	Knowledge base
Objectives	Conceptual structures of a domain	Particular states of a domain
Consistency	Facts always true	Facts true for a particular state of affairs
Actions	Communication	Problem solving
Knowledge	Domain knowledge	Operational knowledge and restricted domain knowledge
Applicability	Shared by community	Specific to system

Note The use of ontologies over knowledge bases for the agent's operational knowledge has also been proposed [Guarino00, Hadzic08]

- The ontologies designed through support of data models are usually **specialized ontologies** and not general ontologies. The number of applications for which these specialized ontologies can be used is limited.

The integration of ontologies with data models into a **unified meta-model** can result in an **effective combination of data, documents and formal knowledge**. This enriches both the data models and increases expressiveness of the domain under analysis. This will help support interoperability between different data bases and bridge heterogeneity issues.

3.8 W3C—The Strong Metadata Modeling Promoter

This approach started with Tim Berners-Lee, who proposed the World Wide Web (WWW) concept in 1989. This concept has been strongly supported by the World Wide Web Consortium (W3C) team since 1992. The W3C mission is to help standardize the semantic web development by proposing useful protocols and guidelines. The aim is to aid long-term web growth and reap its full potential usage [Fensel03]. Since 1999 W3C has proposed more than 110 recommendations, providing the basis for open-forums and discussions. The basic requirement for the web to succeed is to have compatible web technologies provided by different vendors. This requirement, from the W3C point of view, is *"web interoperability."* In theory, with support from powerful web languages and protocols, this requirement would avoid web market fragmentation.

The first metadata language proposed by the W3C is the XML (Extensible Markup Language). It lets users mark up and define data constructs in their own ways. In this way it facilitates sharing of pre-defined structured data across different information systems, particularly over the Internet [Bray04]. XML was developed by the XML Working Group (known as the SGML (Standard Generalized Markup Language) Editorial Review Board originally) that was formed under the W3C in 1996. The design goals of XML include [Fensel03]:

 (i)   *usable over the Internet.*
 (ii) *XML shall support a wide variety of applications.*
 (iii) *XML shall be compatible with SGML.*
 (iv) *It shall be easy to write programs that process XML documents.*
  (v) *The number of optional features in XML is to be kept to the absolute minimum, ideally zero.*
 (vi) *XML documents should be human-legible and reasonably clear.*
(vii) *The XML design should be prepared quickly.*
(viii) *The design of XML shall be formal and concise.*
 (ix) *XML documents shall be easy to create.*
  (x) *Terseness in XML markup is of minimal importance.*

XML allows users to structure data with regard to their content rather than their presentation [Yergeua04]. This is behavioral in nature and provides the tool to map tacit knowledge into explicit knowledge. From this viewpoint, it is different from other metadata systems such as the UML. With XML, large amounts of data can be analyzed, diagnosed, seen, and understood by both humans and machines. Thus XML is useful for ontological construction because, according to Gruber [Gruber93a], an ontology is the explicit specification of a conceptualization, which should be human-understandable and machine process-able. XML, which limits and controls the vocabularies and namespaces, provides the *first level* of metadata.

The following is a simple example of XML annotation: <price currency = "HKD">100</price>. In this example, however, the labels do not bear any meaning for machines but bear meaning for humans. To reduce such limitations, W3C came up with a better solution—XML schema. The XML schema provides structured descriptions for XML documents, which typically are expressed in terms of constraints on the structure and content of documents of that type, above and beyond the basic syntax constraints imposed by XML itself. As an example, it can specify that the content of a "price" label should be a rational number. An XML schema provides a view of the document type at a relatively high level of abstraction. The basic XML is poor in data type specification. For example, the schema does not help specify the meaning of tags, despite the feature to build hierarchies of element types. This hierarchy contains no conceptual knowledge, but only functions as a syntactic shortcut to allow reuse of complex definitions. A naïve way of relating the ontology with XML documents is to match the labels in a XML document syntactically with the names of concepts/properties in the ontology that are associated with it. However the role the data fulfils in the XML document is not clear. Referring to the previous example <price currency = "HKD">100</price>, it is not yet clear whether "price" is the data type of "100", or the value of price is "100". For reliable use on the Semantic Web, it is necessary to interpret data and its type unambiguously. This inspired the emergence of the RDF metadata model to support unambiguous data interpretation, followed by the more advanced version OWL.

3.9 The Web is an Information Treasure Trove

The web is a worldly information treasure trove, but it contains unorganized knowledge in an intertwined fashion. Usually the meaning and importance of a piece of web information depends on subjective interpretations by the potential users. To benefit a community, subjective interpretations should depend on collective agreements—the prelude to consensus certification. The first logical step to reap the potential usefulness of web sources is to organize them into a standard (i.e. community/domain) repertoire. The organization involves: view definitions for terms, attributes, concepts and the associations, classification or categorization of these definitions (sub-ontologies). This is followed by the construction of the corresponding subsumption hierarchy to layout the interconnection among the sub-ontologies. This hierarchy should finally be agreed by consensus to become the "community, domain or enterprise" ontology, which could be made into a machine-usable form. The ontology approach makes the web semantics potentially usable, and from the user's point of view, the web is now semantic (i.e. meanings can be easily extracted and used—semantic web). If one could transform the subsumption hierarchy in the web ontology into a Petri net, then every network/semantic/operation path (in the Petri net) would have a meaning (semantic). Then, tracing such a path for a set of parameters is a logical process or inference. The final path traced out by the inference process is the logical conclusion for the given set of parameters. The connotation of every distinctive semantic path can be predefined in the specific context via a consensus certification process.

The UMLS [UMLS] is a real-life example of how the concept of ontology is realized successfully in the area of Western/allopathic medicine. The UMLS is organized into three layers: (i) the allopathic context, from a specific angle, into the bottom-layer ontology; (ii) the middle-layer semantic net to logically represent the bottom ontology for machine processing; it is the machine process-able form and the processor is the logical parser; and (iii) the top-layer syntactical representation of the semantic net so that human users can formulate the corresponding queries. In fact, all three layers connote the same knowledge in different forms for different purposes. The knowledge, however, must be represented formally and in a retrievable form for practical use. The representation or retrieval form can be a metadata system (e.g. XML). For production systems the meta-system may be converted into technology-oriented databases (e.g. Microsoft (MS) relational database—SQL server) so that tools from different vendors are readily applicable. In this way the chance of premature obsolescence is prevented because the databases are tied in with the related proprietary artefacts of data interoperability. This also applies to the metadata systems; for example, XML, RDF and OWL have less chance of obsolescence because they are supported by the influential W3C and many vendors (e.g. IBM and Microsoft).

As the semantic web keeps developing [Fensel03], its knowledge content is becoming richer and more useful. As a result it should be managed to the benefit of mankind on a global scale. Tim Berners-Lee actually envisioned the semantic web as the natural evolution from the current web. Its evolution involves additions of machine-readable information and automated services. Berners-Lee thought that explicit representations of semantics underlying the web data, programs, pages, and other web resources would support qualitative new services [Fensel03].

3.10   Some Insight into RDF and OWL

Both RDF and OWL are frequently used to implement ontologies and we briefly discuss them here.

Resource Description Framework (RDF) was proposed by W3C as a more formal format for making assertions and leveraging the XML format to represent and transport information. It is a language specifically designed for representing resources and information in the World Wide Web. It is a metadata system extended from the XML, and it clearly defines the details of web resources; for example, title, author, web page modification date, copyright, licensing information of a web document, and/or the availability schedule for sharing resources.

By providing a common framework/infrastructure/standard, the RDF facilitates encoding, exchanging and reusing structured data in the metadata system. Information exchanged via the RDF would have intact meaning. On top of the RDF platform there are many commercial support tools by various vendors. But, the RDF standard makes the data handled by different tools *interoperable*. The obvious RDF advantage for the application designers is the availability of common RDF parsers and processing tools; simply selecting and adopting them. These tools usually recognize items with web identifiers (known as the Uniform Resource Identifiers, or URIs) that describe resources in terms of their simple properties and values.

The hierarchy in Fig. 3.3 lists the following:

(i)   Resource: http://www.ontoweb.com/ ~ test
(ii)   Property: The element <author>
(iii)   Value: The string "Jackei Wong"

The RDF is a generally syntax-independent model for representing resources and their corresponding descriptions, as shown in Fig. 3.4. (The model can be expressed in XML, and the specification uses XML as its syntax for encoding metadata). RDF provides an enhanced representation over XML in defining the relationship such as the concept of class and subclass, and also the triple (Resource, Property, Value) or (Subject, Predicate, Object). RDF is extensible, which means that descriptions can be enriched with additional descriptive information, as shown in Fig. 3.4 (Fig. 3.5).

Although RDF is generally syntax-independent, it provides an XML syntax called serialization syntax. The following is an example:

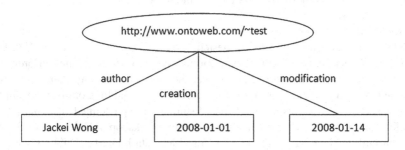

Fig. 3.3 The hierarchy of items within the http URI

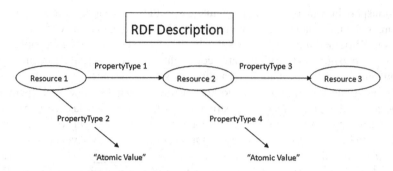

Fig. 3.4 RDF description of resources

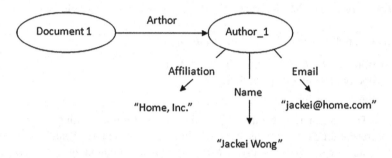

Fig. 3.5 Extensible RDF representation

```
<?xml version"1.0"?>
<RDF>
        <Description about=http://www.ontoweb.com/~test>
                <author>Jackei Wong</author>
                <created>2008-01-01</created>
                <modified>2008-01-14</modified>
        </Description>
</RDF>
```

RDF metadata can be inserted or nested into XML code or vice versa. Yet, for information operability, RDF metadata formats have to be pre-defined in order to facilitate correct information exchange over the web anytime, anywhere and with anyone that operates with the same "format core". The Dublin Core is an example in which a set of properties for describing documents are predefined. The first set of Dublin Core property was defined at the Metadata Workshop in Dublin, Ohio 1995. It is currently maintained by the Dublin Core Metadata Initiative. Dublin Core is a standard for cross-domain information resource description. It provides a simple and standardized set of conventions for describing things online in ways that make them easier to find. It is widely used to describe materials such as video, sound,

Table 3.8 Original 15 elements in simple dublin core

Elements	Definition
Contributor	An entity responsible for making contributions to the content of the resource
Coverage	The extent or scope of the content of the resource
Creator	An entity primarily responsible for making the content of the resource
Format	The physical of digital manifestation of the resource
Date	A date of an event in the lifecycle of the resource
Description	An account of the content of the resource
Identifier	An unambiguous reference to the resource within a given context
Language	A language of the intellectual content of the resource
Publisher	An entity responsible for making the resource available
Relation	A reference to a related resource
Rights	Information about rights held in and over the resource
Source	A reference to a resource from which the present resource is derived
Subject	A topic of the content of the resource
Title	A name given to the resource
Type	The nature of genre of the content of the resource

(reproduced from http://www.w3schools.com/rdf/rdf_dublin.asp)

image, text, as well as those composite media like web pages. Implementations with support from the Dublin Core typically work with both XML and RDF. Simple Dublin Core consists of the following 15 metadata elements [W3Schools] (Table 3.8).

Conceptually the elements in Simple Dublin Core could be construed as pre-defined "data types". In contrast, the XML has only one data type "string". After the original 15 elements specification, refinement of the Dublin Core Metadata Element Set (DCMES) continued. Additional terms were identified by working groups in the Dublin Core Metadata Initiative (DCMI) and judged by the DCMI Usage Board to be in conformance with principles of good practice for the qualification of Dublin Core metadata elements.

RDF element refinements narrow its meaning, and a refined element shares the meaning of the unqualified element but with a more restricted scope. In addition to element refinements, Qualified Dublin Core includes a set of recommended encoding schemes, designed to aid the interpretation of an element value. The schemes include controlled terms and formal notations or parsing rules. A value expressed using an encoding scheme may thus be a token selected from a controlled vocabulary, or a string formatted in accordance with a formal notation. For example, "2008-03-10" can be used as the standard expression of a date. DCMI also maintains a small, general vocabulary recommended for use within the element Type. This vocabulary currently consists of 12 terms. In effect, the refinement is a standardization process. An example of RDF and XML namespace is shown below. An XML namespace is used to unambiguously identify the schema for the Dublin Core terms by pointing to the definitive Dublin Core resource that defines the corresponding semantics. In this example, RDF is nested inside XML—the two are interoperable.

```
<?xml version="1.0"?>
<rdf:RDF
    xmlns:rdf=http://www.w3.org/1999/02/22-rdf-syntax-ns#
    xmlns:dc=http://purl.org/dc/elements/1.1>
            <rdf:Description rdf:about=http://uri-of-Document-1>
                    <dc:creator>Jackei Wong</dc:creator>
            </rdf:Description>
</rdf:RDF>
```

Another example using description element is shown below:

```
<?xml version="1.0"?>
<rdf:RDF
    xmlns:rdf=http://www.w3.org/1999/02/22-rdf-syntax-ns#
    xmlns:cd=http://www.recshop.fake/cd>
            <rdf:Description

    rdf:about=http://www.recshop.fake/cd/Empire_Burlesque>
            <cd:artist>Bob Dylan</cd:artist>
            <cd:country>USA</cd:country>
            <cd:company>Columbia</cd:company>
        </rdf:Description>
</rdf:RDF>
```

RDF is a formalism suitable for metadata annotation; it is a way to work with XML harmoniously. But, it does not provide the special meanings to some terms such as subClassOf of Type. The definitions of these terms rely on the RDF Schema (RDFS), which allows users to define the terms and their associations or relationships. The definitions provide "extra meanings" to particular RDF predicates and resources. The "extra meaning" or semantics specifies how a term should be interpreted. In RDFS, terms include Class, Property, type, subClassOf, range, domain etc. Some examples are as follows:

   (i)   <Person, type, Class>
  (ii)   The type of "Person" is a "Class"
 (iii)   <Professor, subClassOf, Person>
  (iv)   "Professor" is a subclass of the class "Person"
   (v)   <Allan, type, Professor>
  (vi)   The type of "Allan" is a "Professor"
 (vii)   <hasColleague, domain, Person>
(viii)   The domain of "hasColleague" is "Person"

The RDF, however, has some problems as follows:

(i) No distinction between classes and instances (individuals).
(ii) No localized range and domain constraints.
(iii) No existence/cardinality constraints.
(iv) No transitive, inverse or symmetrical properties.
(v) Too weak to describe resources in sufficient detail.
(vi) Difficult to provide reasoning support.

Meanwhile, a powerful web ontology language is expected to have some basic qualities, namely:

(i) It extends existing Web standards (E.g. XML, RDF, RDFS).
(ii) It is easy to use and understand.
(iii) It is formal.
(iv) It has adequate expressive power.
(v) It can provide automated reasoning support.

The few web ontology languages developed after RDF include:

(i) OIL—European researchers
(ii) DAML-ONT—US researchers in DARPA DAML programme
(iii) DAML+OIL—Joint EU/US Committee on Agent Markup Languages and extended RDF
(iv) OWL—W3C—Web-ontology working Group and based on DAML+OIL

The OWL was proposed after the RDF by W3C; the annotations of web semantics have evolved from XML, through RDF to OWL. These three cognate metadata systems are interoperable and nested in one another. OWL basically compensates the RDF shortcomings. It is a family of knowledge representation languages for authoring ontology constructs, and it is endorsed by the W3C. It is also a family of languages based on two (largely, but not entirely, compatible) systems: OWL DL and OWL Lite. Again these two systems are based on Description Logics [Horrocks04], which have attractive and well-understood computational properties. The OWL Full uses a novel semantic model, intended to have compatibility with RDF Schema. OWL ontology constructs are usually serialized using RDF/XML syntax. The W3C-endorsed OWL specification includes the definition of three variants of OWL, with different levels of expressiveness:

(i) OWL Lite—This is a subset of OWL DL and supports classification hierarchy and simple constraints; for example it only permits cardinality values of 0 or 1.
(ii) OWL DL—This supports maximum expressiveness, computational completeness, decidability; it includes all language constructs; its functions correspond with Description Logics (a fragment of FOL (First Order Logic)).
(iii) OWL Full—This supports maximum expressiveness, syntactic freedom of RDF, no computational guarantees; it is the union of OWL syntax and RDF; its reasoning software cannot support complete logical reasoning.

Table 3.9 Comparing RDF, DAML+OIL and OWL

| | Data types | | Types of properties | | Property element | | Classes | |
	Primitive data-type	Numeric min, max	Transitive	Inverse	Import element	Individual element	Negation/disjoint classes	Inheritance
RDF(S)	No	No	No	No	No	Yes	No	Yes
DAML+OIL	Yes	Yes	Yes	Yes	No	Yes	Yes	Yes
OWL	Yes	Yes	Yes	Yes	Yes	Yes	Yes	Yes

Every one of the following sublanguages is a syntactic extension of their simpler predecessors. But, it should be noted that relationship may not be transitive; for example, the following set of relations hold but their inverses do not:

(i)   *Every legal OWL Lite ontology is a legal OWL DL ontology.*
(ii) *Every legal OWL DL ontology is a legal OWL Full ontology.*
(iii) *Every valid OWL Lite conclusion is a valid OWL DL conclusion.*
(iv) *Every valid OWL DL conclusion is a valid OWL Full conclusion.*

In the sequel, a few main OWL characteristics are shown here by the following examples below. Further information can be found at: http://www.w3.org/2004/OWL.

Table 3.9 compares RDF, DAML+OIL and OWL in terms of 8 attributes (e.g. transitive). XML is the 1st-level metadata that contains no meaning for machines but does have meaning to humans. RDF is a metadata system extended from the XML, and it can clearly define the details of web resources (e.g. title, author, web page modification date, copyright, licensing information of a web document, and/or the availability schedule for sharing resources). We can compare RDF and OWL qualitatively in three areas:

(i)   *Data types*—RDF does not contain primitive data-type nor the numeric minimum or maximum functions, but OWL does. *Types of relationship*—No transitive and inverse relationships can be found when using RDF but OWL can have them.
(ii) *Property elements*—Only OWL can import elements into it while RDF cannot. Both of them can set the property of elements individually.
(iii) *Classes*—OWL contains the classes of negation and disjoint while RDF does not. Both of them have the property of class inheritance.

3.11 Transformation of Markup Languages

Figure 3.6 shows the transformation of markup languages (ML) in the course of time. A ML makes use a set of annotations to describe the structure of text, and its layout format. In fact, ML of different forms has been used for decades; for example, computer typesetting and word-processing systems use markup languages.

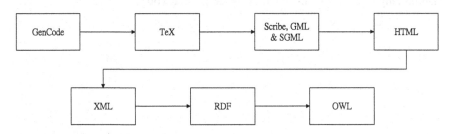

Fig. 3.6 Transformation of markup languages

The idea of "markup languages" was first presented by publishing executive William W. Tunnicliffe at a conference in 1967; it was called "generic coding" at the time. He then led the development of a standard called "GenCode" for the publication industry. In later years, Donald Knuth created another major publishing standard—TeX, and kept continuously refining it in 1970s and 1980s. The focus of TeX is on the detailed layout of text and the font description in order to typeset mathematical books of professional quality. TeX requires considerable skill from the users, so that it is mainly used in the academic area. It is the de facto standard in many scientific disciplines. LaTeX, a TeX macro package, provides a descriptive markup system on top of Tex and is widely used in academic and technical publications (e.g. Springer Verlag).

Scribe, developed by Brian Reid in 1980, is the first language to make a clean and clear distinction between presentation and structure. It was revolutionary at that time because it introduced the idea of styles to be separated from the marked up document, as well as using grammar to control the usage of descriptive elements. It also influenced the development of Generalized Markup Language (GML), and later Standard Generalized Markup Language (SGML), and is a direct ancestor of HTML and LaTeX.

In the early 1980s, SGML was created for the idea that the markup operation should be focused on the structural aspects of a document, with the visual presentation of that structure left to the interpreter. SGML was developed by a committee chaired by Goldfarb. It incorporated ideas from many different sources including Tunnicliffe's project, GenCode. SGML specified a syntax which includes the markup in documents, and it separately describes what and where the tags are allowed (Document Type Definition (DTD) or schema). This syntax allows authors to create and use any markup they want, or select tags that make the most sense in their own languages. So, SGML is recognized as a proper meta-language from which other markup languages are derived.

Tim Berners-Lee learned SGML and used its syntax to create HyperText Markup Language (HTML), which is similar to other SGML-based tag languages, but much simpler. However, some computer scientists disputed that HTML was hard to use because it restricts the tag placement. These scientists argued that easy-to-use markup languages should be hierarchical instead of being just a *language of container*". The hierarchical argument led to the emergence of other languages such as XML and its interoperable partners including RDF and OWL. The contemporary markup languages follow the "what you see is what you get" style.

3.12 OWL Language

In this section we discuss some of the features of the OWL ontology language.

OWL – Headers
<owl:Ontology rdf:about="">
■ Ontology name
<rdfs:comment>An example OWL ontology</rdfs:comment>
<owl:priorVersion   rdf:resource="http://www.w3.org/TR/2003/PR-owl-guide-20031215/wine"/>
■ Ontology versioning
<owl:imports   rdf:resource="http://www.w3.org/TR/2004/REC-owl-guide-20040210/food"/>
■ Import other ontologies
<rdfs:label>Wine Ontology</rdfs:label>
■ Natural language label

OWL – Classes
<owl:Class rdf:ID="PotableLiquid"/>
<owl:Class   rdf:ID="http://www.w3.org/TR/2004/REC-owl-guide-20040210/wine#Region" />

<owl:Class rdf:ID="Wine">
  <rdfs:subClassOf rdf:resource="&food;PotableLiquid"/>
  <rdfs:label xml:lang="en">wine</rdfs:label>
  <rdfs:label xml:lang="fr">vin</rdfs:label>

  ...
</owl:Class>

OWL – Individuals
<Region rdf:ID="CentralCoastRegion" />

<owl:Thing rdf:ID="CentralCoastRegion" />
<owl:Thing rdf:about="#CentralCoastRegion">
  <rdf:type rdf:resource="#Region"/>
</owl:Thing>

■ "CentralCoastRegion" is a *member* of "Region"

A more detailed example illustrating the properties of OWL is given in Appendix 2.

3.13 Recapitulation

In this chapter, the features and existing definitions of an Ontology as a means for providing shared.

Next we discussed the following uses of the Ontology namely:

- Strong and Unambiguous Communication Mechanism through the use of a shared unified knowledge representation
- Ontology Mediated Information Access to Databases or Information repositories which might have different data models or formats
- Ontology and Semantic Web Services to allow a decoupled approach to service creation and utilization
- Ontology Based Multi Agent Systems where ontologies provide the shared knowledge base for the multi Agents

These uses of an Ontology could be helpful for building an Intelligent TCM Telemedicine System. In the next chapter, we utilize the Ontology paradigm for building the Intelligent TCM System.

Appendix 1

A summary of the Ontology Modelling Notation is given here:

		Partition classes *Y1*, *Y2* and *Y3*.
Data type property		Data type property *Y* which is functional and its type is string.
		Class *X* has data type property *Y* which is functional and its type is string.
Object property		Object property *A* which is non-functional.
		Class *X* has relations with class *Y*. The relation considers as an object property named *A* which is non-functional property.
Property characteristic		
- Functional property		A functional property *X*.
- Non-functional property		A non-functional property *X*.
- Inverse functional property		An inverse functional property *X*.
- Symmetric property		A symmetric property *X*.
- Transitive property		A transitive property *X*.
Property restriction		

Concept/Term	Notation	Semantics
Class	<<Concept>> X	Ontology class *X*.
owl-Thing Class	<<Concept>> Thing	All classes in ontology are subclasses of class *owl:Thing*.
Generalisation	△	To express either class-subclass or property-sub property.
	<<Concept>> X △ <<Concept>> Y	Class *Y* is a subclass of class *X*.
	<<Object property>> Y1 △ <<Object property>> Y2	Object property *Y2* is sub property of object property *Y1*.
	<<Concept>> X △ disjoint — <<Concept>> Y1 <<Concept>> Y2 <<Concept>> Y3	Disjoint classes *Y1*, *Y2* and *Y3*.
	<<Concept>> X △ decomposition — <<Concept>> Y1 <<Concept>> Y2 <<Concept>> Y3	Decomposed classes *Y1*, *Y2* and *Y3*.

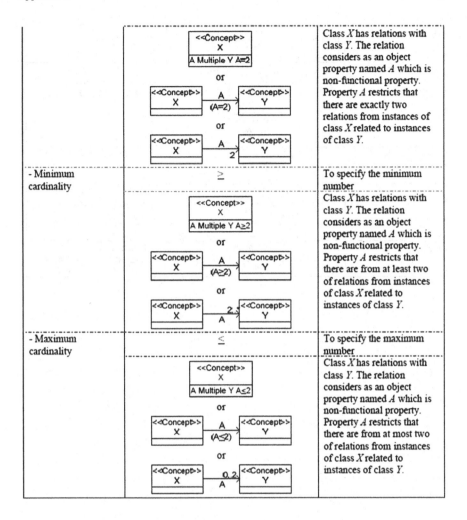

	$$\text{<<Concept>>}$$ X A Multiple Y A=2 or <<Concept>> X — A (A=2) — <<Concept>> Y or <<Concept>> X — A 2 — <<Concept>> Y	Class X has relations with class Y. The relation considers as an object property named A which is non-functional property. Property A restricts that there are exactly two relations from instances of class X related to instances of class Y.
- Minimum cardinality	$\geq$	To specify the minimum number
	<<Concept>> X A Multiple Y A≥2 or <<Concept>> X — A (A≥2) — <<Concept>> Y or <<Concept>> X — 2..* A — <<Concept>> Y	Class X has relations with class Y. The relation considers as an object property named A which is non-functional property. Property A restricts that there are from at least two of relations from instances of class X related to instances of class Y.
- Maximum cardinality	$\leq$	To specify the maximum number
	<<Concept>> X A Multiple Y A≤2 or <<Concept>> X — A (A≤2) — <<Concept>> Y or <<Concept>> X — 0..2 A — <<Concept>> Y	Class X has relations with class Y. The relation considers as an object property named A which is non-functional property. Property A restricts that there are from at most two of relations from instances of class X related to instances of class Y.

Annotation property		Class X has annotation property.
Association class		Class A is association class of object property related class X to class Y.
Class instance		a is instance of class A.
Property instance		a is instance of property A and b is an instance of property B.
oneOf		Functional data type property A relates to a set of data value of 'a', 'b' and 'c'.

Appendix 2

We give a more detailed example using OWL to illustrate some of its properties here.

OWL – Namespace
```
<rdf:RDF
xmlns=http://www.w3.org/TR/2004/REC-owl-guide-20040210/wine#
xmlns:vin=http://www.w3.org/TR/2004/REC-owl-guide-20040210/wine#
xmlns:food=http://www.w3.org/TR/2004/REC-owl-guide-20040210/food#
xmlns:owl=http://www.w3.org/2002/07/owl#
xmlns:rdf=http://www.w3.org/1999/02/22-rdf-syntax-ns#
xmlns:rdfs=http://www.w3.org/2000/01/rdf-schema#
xmlns:xsd=http://www.w3.org/2001/XMLSchema#>
```

OWL – Headers
```
<owl:Ontology rdf:about="">
```
- Ontology name
```
<rdfs:comment>An example OWL ontology</rdfs:comment>
<owl:priorVersion   rdf:resource="http://www.w3.org/TR/2003/PR-owl-guide-
20031215/wine"/>
```
- Ontology versioning
```
<owl:imports        rdf:resource="http://www.w3.org/TR/2004/REC-owl-guide-
20040210/food"/>
```
- Import other ontologies
```
<rdfs:label>Wine Ontology</rdfs:label>
```
- Natural language label

OWL – Classes
```
<owl:Class rdf:ID="PotableLiquid"/>
<owl:Class              rdf:ID="http://www.w3.org/TR/2004/REC-owl-guide-
20040210/wine#Region" />
<owl:Class rdf:ID="Wine">
  <rdfs:subClassOf rdf:resource="&food;PotableLiquid"/>
  <rdfs:label xml:lang="en">wine</rdfs:label>
  <rdfs:label xml:lang="fr">vin</rdfs:label>

  ...
</owl:Class>
```

OWL – Individuals
```
<Region rdf:ID="CentralCoastRegion" />

<owl:Thing rdf:ID="CentralCoastRegion" />
<owl:Thing rdf:about="#CentralCoastRegion">
   <rdf:type rdf:resource="#Region"/>
</owl:Thing>
```

■   "CentralCoastRegion" is a *member* of "Region"

OWL - Properties
```
<owl:Class rdf:ID="WineDescriptor" />
<owl:Class rdf:ID="WineColor">
   <rdfs:subClassOf rdf:resource="#WineDescriptor" />
   ...
</owl:Class>

<owl:ObjectPropertyrdf:ID="hasWineDescriptor">
   <rdfs:domain rdf:resource="#Wine" />
   <rdfs:range rdf:resource="#WineDescriptor" />
</owl:ObjectProperty>

<owl:ObjectProperty rdf:ID="hasColor">
   <rdfs:subPropertyOf rdf:resource="#hasWineDescriptor" />
   <rdfs:range rdf:resource="#WineColor" />
   ...
</owl:ObjectProperty>

<owl:Class rdf:ID="Vintage">
   <rdfs:subClassOf>
     <owl:Restriction>
       <owl:onProperty rdf:resource="#vintageOf"/>
```

```
        <owl:minCardinality rdf:datatype="&xsd;nonNegativeInteger">
          1</owl:minCardinality>
      </owl:Restriction>
    </rdfs:subClassOf>
</owl:Class>

<owl:ObjectProperty rdf:ID="vintageOf">
  <rdfs:domain rdf:resource="#Vintage" />
  <rdfs:range rdf:resource="#Wine" />
</owl:ObjectProperty>
```

OWL – Datatype Properties
```
<owl:Class rdf:ID="VintageYear" />
<owl:DatatypeProperty rdf:ID="yearValue">
  <rdfs:domain rdf:resource="#VintageYear" />
  <rdfs:range rdf:resource="&xsd;positiveInteger"/>
</owl:DatatypeProperty>

<VintageYear rdf:ID="Year1998">
  <yearValue rdf:datatype="&xsd;positiveInteger">1998
    </yearValue>
</VintageYear>
```

OWL – Transitive Property
- $P(x,y)$ and $P(y,z)$ implies $P(x,z)$

```
<owl:ObjectProperty rdf:ID="locatedIn">
  <rdf:type rdf:resource="&owl;TransitiveProperty" />
  <rdfs:domain rdf:resource="&owl;Thing" />
  <rdfs:range rdf:resource="#Region" />
</owl:ObjectProperty>

<Region rdf:ID="SantaCruzMountainsRegion">
  <locatedIn rdf:resource="#CaliforniaRegion" />
</Region>

<Region rdf:ID="CaliforniaRegion">
  <locatedIn rdf:resource="#USRegion" />
</Region>
```

OWL – Inverse Property
- $P_1(x,y) \rightarrow P_2(y,x)$

```
<owl:ObjectProperty rdf:ID="IsTaughtBy">
```

```
    <rdf:type rdf:resource="&owl;InverseProperty" />
    <rdfs:domain rdf:resource="#Teacher" />
    <rdfs:range rdf:resource="#Teacher" />
</owl:ObjectProperty>
```

OWL – Symmetric Property
■ P(x,y) iff P(y,x)

```
<owl:ObjectProperty rdf:ID="adjacentRegion">
    <rdf:type rdf:resource="&owl;SymmetricProperty" />
    <rdfs:domain rdf:resource="#Region" />
    <rdfs:range rdf:resource="#Region" />
</owl:ObjectProperty>
```

```
<Region rdf:ID="MendocinoRegion">
    <locatedIn rdf:resource="#CaliforniaRegion" />
    <adjacentRegion rdf:resource="#SonomaRegion" />
</Region>
```

OWL – Functional Property
■ P(x,y) and P(x,z) implies y=z

```
<owl:Class rdf:ID="VintageYear" />
<owl:ObjectProperty rdf:ID="hasVintageYear">
    <rdf:type rdf:resource="&owl;FunctionalProperty" />
    <rdfs:domain rdf:resource="#Vintage" />
    <rdfs:range rdf:resource="#VintageYear" />
</owl:ObjectProperty>
```

OWL – Property Restriction
```
<owl:Class rdf:ID="Wine">
    <rdfs:subClassOf rdf:resource="&food;PotableLiquid" />
    ...
    <rdfs:subClassOf>
      <owl:Restriction>
        <owl:onProperty rdf:resource="#hasMaker" />
        <owl:allValuesFrom rdf:resource="#Winery" />
      </owl:Restriction>
    </rdfs:subClassOf>
    ...
</owl:Class>
```

■ allValuesFrom: For all wines, if they have makers, all the makers are wineries
■ someValuesFrom: For all wines, they have at least one maker that is a winery

```
<owl:Class rdf:ID="Vintage">
  <rdfs:subClassOf>
    <owl:Restriction>
      <owl:onProperty rdf:resource="#hasVintageYear"/>
      <owl:cardinality rdf:datatype="&xsd;nonNegativeInteger">1
        </owl:cardinality>
    </owl:Restriction>
  </rdfs:subClassOf>
</owl:Class>
```

- Every Vintage has exactly one VintageYear

OWL – Ontology Mapping
- To show a particular class or property in one ontology is *equivalent* to a class or property in a second ontology

```
<owl:Class rdf:ID="Wine">
  <owl:equivalentClass rdf:resource="&vin;Wine"/>
</owl:Class>
```

```
<owl:Class rdf:ID="TexasThings">
  <owl:equivalentClass>
    <owl:Restriction>
      <owl:onProperty rdf:resource="#locatedIn" />
      <owl:someValuesFrom rdf:resource="#TexasRegion" />
    </owl:Restriction>
  </owl:equivalentClass>
</owl:Class>
```

```
<Wine rdf:ID="MikesFavoriteWine">
  <owl:sameAs rdf:resource="#StGenevieveTexasWhite" />
</Wine>
```

OWL – Complex Classes
- OWL supports the basic set operations, namely *union*, *intersection* and *complement*

```
<owl:Class rdf:ID="WhiteWine">
  <owl:intersectionOf rdf:parseType="Collection">
    <owl:Class rdf:about="#Wine" />
    <owl:Restriction>
      <owl:onProperty rdf:resource="#hasColor" />
      <owl:hasValue rdf:resource="#White" />
```

```
        </owl:Restriction>
      </owl:intersectionOf>
    </owl:Class>

    <owl:Class rdf:ID="Fruit">
      <owl:unionOf rdf:parseType="Collection">
        <owl:Class rdf:about="#SweetFruit" />
        <owl:Class rdf:about="#NonSweetFruit" />
      </owl:unionOf>
    </owl:Class>
```

From the examples above, it becomes obvious that the OWL is more powerful than RDF, which is more expressive than the preceding XML.

References

[Alonso04]   Alonso, G., Casati, F., Kuno, H., Machiraju, V.: Web Services: Concepts, Architectures and Applications. Springer, Heidelberg (2004)

[Berners01]   Berners-Lee, T., James, H., Ora, L.: The semantic web. Sci. Am. Mag. **284**, 28–37 (2001)

[Bray04]   Bray, T., Paoli, J., Sperberg-McQueen, C.M., Maler, E., Yergeua, F.: Extensible markup language (XML) 1.0—origin and goals, 4th edn. World Wide Web Consortium (2004)

[Chang06]   Chang, E., Dillon, T., Hussain, F.K.: Trust and Reputation for Service Oriented Environment: Technologies for Building Business Intelligence and Consumer Confidence. Wiley, New York (2006)

[Clark05]   Clark, D.: Position Paper for Rules Concerning Project Management Ontologies Rule Languages for Interoperability, W3C (2005)

[Coplien04]   Coplien, J.: Organizational patterns: beyond technology to people. In: Proceedings of the 6th International Conference on Enterprise Information Systems (ICES2004), Porto, Portugal (2004)

[Corazzon04]   Corazzon, R.: Descriptive and formal ontology—a resource guide to contemporary research. http://www.formalontology.it/ (2004)

[Denny04]   Denny, M.: Ontology tools survey. http://ww.xml.com/lpt/a/2004/07/14/onto.html (2004)

[Dhesiaseelan04] Dhesiaseelan, A., Ragunathan, V.: Web Services Container Reference Architecture (WSCRA), ICWS04 (2004)

[Dillon93]   Dillon, T.S.: Object Oriented Conceptual Modeling. Prentice Hall, New Jersey (1993)

[Dillon07a]   Dillon, T.S., Wu, C., Chang, E.: Reference architectural styles for service-oriented computing, keynote. In: IFIP NPC. Dalian, China (2007)

[Dillon07b]   Dillon, T.S., Wu, C., Chang, E.: GRIDSpace: semantic grid services on the web—evolution towards a softgrid, keynote. In: Conference on IEEE Semantics, Knowledge and Grid, Xian, China (2007)

[Dillon08]   Dillon, T.S., Chang, E., Hadzic, M., Wongthongtham, P.: Differentiating conceptual modelling from data modelling, knowledge modelling and ontology modelling and a notation for ontology modelling, pp. 7–17. APCCM (2008)

[Dunn05]   Dunn, C., Hollander, J.: The REA Enterprise Ontology: Value System and Value Chain Modelling, Enterprise Information Systems: A Pattern-based Approach. McGraw Hill, New York (2005)

[Fensel01]   Fensel, D.: Ontologies: Silver Bullet for Knowledge Management and Electronic Commerce. Springer, Heidelberg (2001)

[Fensel03]   Fensel, D.: Ontologies: Silver Bullet for Knowledge Management and Electronic Commerce, 2nd edn. Springer, Berlin (2003)

[Gruber93a]   Gruber, T.R.: A translation approach to portable ontology specification. Knowl. Acquis. **5**(2), 199–220 (1993)

[Gruber93b]   Gruber, T.R.: Toward principles for the design of ontologies used for knowledge sharing. In: Nicola, G., Roberto, P. (eds.) International Workshop on Formal Ontology in Conceptual Analysis and Knowledge Representation. Kluwer Academic Publishers, Deventer (1993)

[Guarino00]   Guarino, N., Welty, C.: Towards a methodology for ontology based model engineering, (2000). http://citseer.ist.psu.edu/b12206.htm

[Hadzic05]   Hadzic, M., Chang, E.: Medical ontologies to support human disease research and control. Int. J. Web Grid Serv. **1**(2), 139–150 (2005)

[Hadzic08]   Hadzic, M., Wongthongtham, P., Chang, E., Dillon, T.S.: Integrated MultiAgent and Ontology Development. Springer, Heidelberg (2008)

[Hamilton02]   Hamilton,J.A.,Rosen,J.,Summers,P.A.:DevelopingInteroperabilityMetrics. Auburn University, USA, (2002). http://www.eng.auburn.edu/users/hamiliton/security/spawar/6_Deveoping_Interoperability_Metrics/pdf

[Hecker08]   Hecker, M., Dillon, T.S., Chang, E.: Privacy ontology support for E-commerce. IEEE Internet Comput. **12**, 54–81 (2008)

[Hecker06]   Hecker, M., Dillon, T.S.: Ontological privacy support for the medical domain. In: eHPass National e-Health Privacy and Security Symposium, Brisbane, Australia (2006)

[Herman08]   Herman, I.: Semantic Web activity statement, W3C, 7 Mar 2008

[Högg06]   Högg, R., Meckel, M., Stanoevska-Slabeva, K., Martignoni, R.: Overview of business models for Web 2.0 communities, GeNeMe (2006)

[Horrocks04]   Horrocks, I., Patel-Schneider, P.F.: Reducing OWL entailment to description logic satisfiability. In: Web Semantics, vol. 1, no. 4 (2004)

[IBM03]   IBM and Sandpiper Software Incorporated, Ontology definition meta-model, http://www.omg.org/docs/ad/05-8-01.pdf (2003). Accessed 14 December 2008

[JWong08b]   Wong, J.H.K., Lin, W.W.K., Wong, A.K.Y., Dillon, T.S.: An ontology supported meta-interface for the development and installation of customized web-based telemedicine systems. In: Proceedings of the 6th IFIP Workshop on Software Technologies for Future Embedded and Ubiquitous Systems (SEUS), Capri Island, Italy, 1–3 Oct 2008

[JWong09b]   Wong, J.H.K., Lin, W.W.K., Wong, A.K.Y.: Enterprise-ontology-driven TCM (Traditional Chinese Medicine) Telemedicine System Generation. In: Proceedings of the 4th International Food—New Horizons in Chinese Medicine and Health Food Symposium, Hong Kong, 29–30 Oct 2009

[JWong09d]   Jackei, H., Wong, K.: Ph.D. thesis: web-based data mining and discovery of useful herbal ingredients (WD^2UHI). Department of Computing, Hong Kong Polytechnic University (2009)

[Klein01]   Klein, M., Fensel, D., van Harmelen, F., Horrocks, I.: The relation
                 between ontologies and XML schemas. In: Link oping Electronic
                 Articles in Computer and Information Science, vol. 6 (2011)
[Lin06]   Lin, K.-J.: Serving Web 2.0 with SOA (keynote presentation). ICEBE,
                 Shanghai, China (2006)
[Lopez99]   Lopez, F.: Overview of methodologies for building ontologies (1999).
                 http://www.ontology.org/maim/presentations/madrid/analysis.pdf
[Noy03]   Noy, N.F., Klein, M.: Ontology evolution: not the same as schema
                 evolution. Knowl. Inf. Syst. **5**, 428–440 (2003)
[Shadbolt06]   Shadbolt, N., Hall, W., Berners-Lee, T.: The semantic web revisited.
                 IEEE Intell. Syst. **21**(3), 96–101 (2006)
[Sidhu06]   Sidhu, A.S., Dillon, T.S., Chang, E.: Integration of protein data sources
                 through PO. In: 17th International Conference on Database and Expert
                 Systems Applications (DEXA 2006), pp. 519–527, Poland (2006)
[Spyns02]   Spyns, P., Meersmen, R., Jarrar, M.: Data modelling versus ontology
                 engineering. ACM SIGMOD Rec. **31**(4), 12–17 (2002)
[Studer98]   Studer, R., Benjamins, V., Fensel, D.: Knowledge engineering: principles
                 and methods. IEEE Trans. Data Knowl. Eng. **25**, 161–97 (1998)
[Taniar06]   Taniar, D., Rahayu, J. (ed.): Web Semantics and Ontology. Idea Group
                 Incorporated, Hershey (2006)
[UMLS]   UMLS: http://umls.nlm.nih.gov/
[W3Cc]   W3C Web site: http://www.w3.org/
[W3Schools]   W3 Schools: http://www.w3schools.com/
[Wongthongtham06a] Wongthongtham, P., Chang, E., Dillon, T.S., Sommerville, I.: Ontology-
                 based multi-site software development methodology and tools. J. Syst.
                 Archit. **52**(11), 640–653 (2006)
[Wongthongtham06b] Wongthongtham, P.: Ontology and Multi-agent-based Systems for
                 Human Disease Studies. Ph.D. thesis, Curtin University (2006)
[Wu07]   Wu, C., Chang, E.: Aligning with the web: an atom-based architecture
                 for web services discovery. Service-Oriented Comput. Appl. **1**, 97–116
                 (2007)
[Yergeua04]   Yergeua, F., Bra, T., Paoli, J., Sperberg-McQueen, S., Maler, E.:
                 Extensible markup language (XML) 1.0, 3rd edn. W3C Recommendation
                 (2004)
[Zhao08]   Zhao, S., Chang, E.J., Dillon, T.S.: Knowledge extraction from web-
                 based application source code: an approach to database reverse
                 engineering for ontology development. In: Proceedings of International
                 Conference on Information Re-use and Integration (IEEE IRI 2008), Las
                 Vegas (2008)

Chapter 4
Ontology for Traditional Chinese Medicine (TCM)

4.1 Introduction

As discussed in Chap. 3, a consensus-certified ontology is useful for passing on knowledge in an unambiguous manner because it contains a standard vocabulary with clearly defined meanings. For a global type of ontology, the number of experts involved in the process of consensus certification process can be very large. The aim is to ensure the ontology achieves final precision. For small ontologies, only a small number of experts may be involved to protect privacy and its proprietary nature. Yet the ultimate aim is the same—to ensure unambiguous communication and unambiguous passing on of knowledge.

Small ontologies are usually skeletal. They are usually built on available classical information already enshrined in canons, treatises and recorded histories, and put together by a process of consensus certification. In this light, the PuraPharm onto-core is a typical skeletal ontology. A skeletal onto-core can bring considerable financial benefits to the owner because of its monopoly nature. All the software systems customized from the same enterprise ontology as the base, wholly or partly, are cognate because they can communicate unambiguously with one another, only restricted by their vocabulary subsets extracted from the master during the customization process. If two ontologies were customized for two different customer specifications, they can still communicate unambiguously but to a lesser degree.

4.2 Usefulness of Ontology in TCM

Our previous research reports indicate that applying an ontology to TCM is very beneficial [JWong08c]. The reason is that the TCM formalisms can be laid out in the ontological blueprint precisely for consensus certification. This can be achieved with the help of an effective specification/modeling language [W3Ca, Taniar06]

© Springer-Verlag Berlin Heidelberg 2015
A.K.Y. Wong et al., *Semantically Based Clinical TCM Telemedicine Systems*,
Studies in Computational Intelligence 587, DOI 10.1007/978-3-662-46024-5_4

like the Ontology Modelling Notation given in Sect. 3.4 and Appendix 1. This would form the basis of a design and implementation model using a modelling language, such as those proposed by the W3C, namely, XML, RDF and OWL [W3Cb] which can help convert the consensus-certified ontology blueprint layout into an operational web-based telemedicine system.

In order to facilitate understanding of these issues, the following practical definitions of an ontology and related ideas will be used in the rest of the book namely:

(a) Ontology—It is the explicit specification of a conceptualization of 3 conceptual levels: the 1st or theoretical level—pure philosophy of a domain and not 100 % implementable in every case; the 2nd local enterprise level—facts in a domain (a subset of the 1st level) that suit the operation of an enterprise and is therefore implementable; and the 3rd local-of-the-local level—variants customized from a predefined enterprise ontology.

(b) Ontology categories—There are at least two main categories: (i) consultative— for the user to familiarize themselves with the domain including facts and conjectures, that is, for passing on communal/domain knowledge unambiguously; and (ii) practical (e.g. TCM clinical practice)—practice with adherence to documented facts only.

(c) Ontology architecture and implementation—This is usually a 3-layer architecture with cross-layer semantic transitivity [JWong09a]: the top layer for human manipulation—this is the query system to reflect exactly the middle layer; middle layer for machine understanding and execution (parsing)—this is the semantic net to exactly reflect the bottom semantic ontology; and the bottom layer for representing the domain knowledge—this includes concepts and lexicon (vocabulary) and their relationships (Fig. 4.1).

The objectives and requirements of any ontology are defined by its creator, but the actual usefulness may far exceed what was previously aimed for. For example, the original aim of the PuraPharm enterprise onto-core was to customize a cognate system that can interact unambiguously over the web. Yet, the prolonged use of the cognate systems revealed that any customized onto-core based system can evolve to help the physician to deliver more accurate diagnosis and effective treatment. The key lies in the general concept of similarity [JWong09a], which may match the specific formalism of a domain as illustrated by the following TCM example. Usually the evolution of an onto-core can happen in two stages. In the first stage the evolution is on-line, and the new knowledge appended to the extant onto-core provides only uncertified opinions to the user. These opinions are based partially on the consensus-certified knowledge in the onto-core and the rest from the newly acquired information, which may be included officially into the master onto-core in the new round of consensus certification. The inclusion of the newly acquired raw information into the master onto-core allows the system to evolve so that it would be part of the future systems customized from the new master.

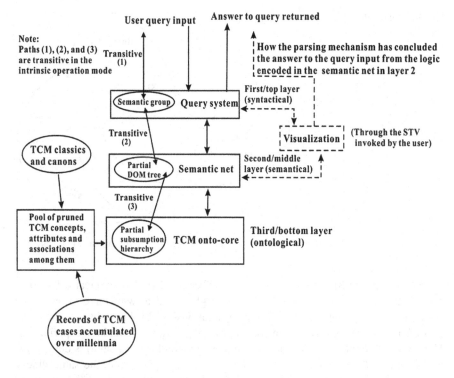

Fig. 4.1 Three layer architecture diagram

4.3 Semantic Aliasing

Useful information can be discovered from the TCM onto-core if some automatic smart algorithms are included in the host system. These smart algorithms should make discoveries based on documented TCM formalisms or principles. For example, the TCM formalism or SIMILARITY/SAME (*SAME and* "同" *are translational synonyms*) principle, is a classical terminology that has been used successfully for making discoveries from the PuraPharm TCM onto-core [JWong09a]. In the Chinese TCM classic this formalism is "同病異治, 異病同治", and it is translated by the World Health Organization in English as: "*If the symptoms are the same or similar, different conditions could be treated in the same way medically, independent of whether they come from the same illness or different ones* [WHO07]."

In fact, rules and principles in a domain form the backbone of the domain knowledge. Through these rules and principles, the correctness of any artifacts constructed for the domain can be verified. In this book, these rules and principles are referred to as axioms; the SIMILARITY/SAME principle in the TCM domain is an axiom.

Fig. 4.2 Automatic semantic aliasing

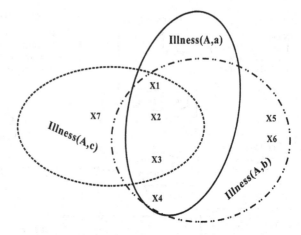

Legend: a, b and c are 3 different geographical regions

The meaning of SIMILARITY/SAME/"同" can be logically explicated by using the example shown in Fig. 4.2. In this example, we deal with three different illnesses or sets and their axiomatic logical relationship. In this light, the three illnesses/subsets are extracted from the illness population by random experiments. The subset Illness (A, a) (i.e. illness A for the geographical region a) is defined by the parameters/attributes X1, X2, X3 and X4; Illness (A, b) (i.e. the same illness name for region b) by X1, X2, X3, X4, X5 and X6; and Illness (A, c) (i.e. the same illness name for region c) by X1, X2, X3, X4 and X7. Let us assume that the prescriptions for Illness (A, a), Illness (A, b) and Illness (A, c) are *PAa*, *PAb* and *PAc* respectively. By applying the classical TCM SIMILARITY/SAME/"同" principle, the total/common set of usable prescriptions for treating the three illnesses should be $P_{all} = PAa \cup PAb \cup PAc$. The $\cup$ operation (i.e. union) axiomatically associates the three different sets of prescriptions into a single pool (i.e. common set P_{all}) by their common attributes/factors (i.e. X1, X2, X3 and X). That is, the three illnesses are defined by the same set of basic parameters but the two sets have additional different attributes on top of the common set, possibly due to geographical and epidemiological differences.

If one arbitrarily takes Illness (A, a) as the ***referential point/host***, then axiomatically Illness (A, b) is *very similar or strongly similar but not logically the same*. From this point of view, the similarity is 4/4 or 1 (as there are 4 entities from the view point of Illness (A, a)—the numerator, and Illness (A, b) contains all 4 entities —the denominator). From Illness (A, b)'s angle, however, Illness (A, a) is only 4/6 or 66.7 % similar because of the different number of defining attributes in the two sets. To generalize two arbitrary sets, S1 and S2 are synonyms (exactly or 100 % the same) only if the axiomatic relationship, $S1 = S2$ holds (i.e. logically equivalent). The probability (P) for the logical expression $P(S1 \cup S2) = P(S1) + P(S2) - P(S1 \cap S2)$ indicates that S1 and S2 are only *aliases* of the resemblance probability (i.e. similarity) equal to $P(S1 \cap S2)$, where $\cup$ and $\cap$ are the logical union and intersection operators respectively. The process of calculating the $P(S1 \cap S2)$ index is called automatic semantic aliasing [JWong08a].

Figure 4.3 shows how automatic semantic aliasing (ASA) would help physicians treat patients more effectively and would lead to discoveries in an on-line fashion. In this example, it is assumed that in the ontology based system, only the Illness (A, a) is defined, consensus-certified, and resident when the system runs with ASA support. If any physician enters through the system interface the symptoms X1, X2, X3 and X4 as the parameters, then the system would unambiguously suggest the resident standard PAa as the only prescription for treatment. Now, if the ASA mechanism in this system is invoked, then it searches the web for TCM cases other than those already recorded in the certified onto-core. If the Illness (A, b) and Illness (A, c) cases are found, they would be included into the extant system onto-core as temporary appendages, in the on-line manner. They are temporary because they have not yet been consensus-certified. The resident ASA mechanism, however, would have axiomatically reasoned the logical relationship $P_{all} = PAa \cup PAb \cup PAc$ on-line. Now if the physician has encountered an unknown illness X of dubious origin x, namely, Illness (X, x) defined by the symptoms X1, X3, X8 and X9, then the ASA would automatically suggest the set of prescriptions P_{all} for its treatment because of the common attributes X1 and X3. Using the consensus-certified Illness (A, a) as the only reference point, the efficacy likelihood of P_{all} is 2/4 or 50 % for Illness (X, x) because the only common attributes shared by Illness

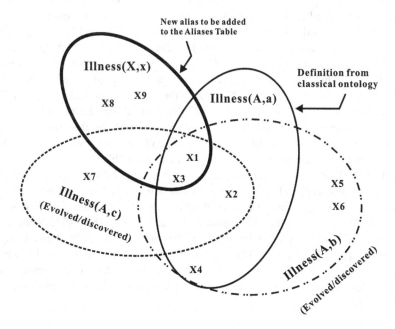

Fig. 4.3 Illness (X, x) is a new alias for the Illness (A, a)

(A, a) and Illness (X, x) are X1 and X3. Yet, P_{all} is a potentially discovery for treating the unknown Illness (X, x) as well as Illness (A, a), Illness (A, b) and Illness (A, c). This new information/opinions suggested by the ASA would be accepted as real discoveries by the community only after they are consensus-certified at a later stage.

Building a useful ontology to support computer/web based operation is no easy task because the corresponding semantic network (or semantic net) must be transitive and logically correct. The initial ontology blueprint layout is usually textual and/or diagrammatic to facilitate human understanding and thus the consensus certification process. The layout should then be translated meticulously into the corresponding semantic network, which is basically a logical subsumption hierarchy [Guarino95]. The original blueprint layout for human understanding and the corresponding semantic net implemented for machine understanding and execution should be logically cross-layer transitive [JWong09d]. That is, any entities in the blueprint layout should be matched by the corresponding entities in the semantic net or vice versa, anytime and anywhere. All the information captured by the layout is eventually stored in the database of choice. When the semantic net is in action, it retrieves the required information as specified by the user in the query entered via the system interface. This query is converted into the form understood by the semantic net by the predefined "*retrieval algorithm* (RA)". For example, the proprietary RA is part of the PuraPharm D/P (diagnosis/prescription) system in Yan Oi Tong (YOT) mobile clinics.

A precise ontology blueprint layout definitely needs the support of an effective tool such as the popular Unified Modeling Language (UML). Figure 4.4 is a mini-ontology conceptualization constructed from a small set of raw clinical data by using UML (Unified Modeling Language) [Kogut02, Dillon14]. In this UML example, ten clinical entities are uniquely identified. In the {0/咳嗽/Cough} entity the unique symbols/identifiers, "0", "咳嗽" and "Cough" have the same meaning (i.e. "0" for machine understanding/"咳嗽" is Chinese/"Cough" is English). Solid-line arcs (e.g. between "3" and "4") mark the logically transitive relationships between the entities at both ends. The physical entities can be placed anywhere within the supporting database but their retrieval depends on the "*retrieval algorithm* (RA)", which should be part of the overall software system. The RA is usually based on predicate logic e.g. if "a" is true then "b".

In light of UML, the aggregation relationship in Fig. 4.4 can be construed as a "*part-of*" relationship, indicating that a "whole" object consists of "*part*" objects [Dillon93, Dillon14]. This kind of relationship exists commonly in XML documents widely adopted by the web operators. For example, {1/風寒襲肺/Wind-Cold Assailing the Lung} is part-of {0/咳嗽/Cough}, and {8/咳嗽聲重/Heavy Cough} is part-of {5/咳嗽/Cough}. The "*part-of*" relationship facilitates high-level semantic visualization (e.g. the ontology blueprint layout for the consensus certification process) before the actual logical implementation into the corresponding semantic net.

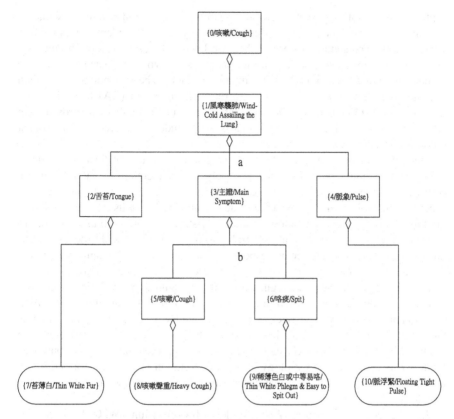

Fig. 4.4 UML organization of raw clinical data

4.4   Choice of Modeling Tools

Choosing an appropriate modeling tool for laying out the ontological blueprint/ scheme in mind would enhance the success of building the final system because this scheme is the basis for the semantic net of the overall computer-aided ontology-based system. Successful examples of such kinds of ontology-based systems include: (a) the UMLS (Unified Medical Language System [UMLS]) developed by the US National Library of Medicine; and (b) the D/P (diagnosis/prescription) system developed by PuraPharm for mobile-clinic operations [JWong08a]. As explained in Chap. 1, from past experience computer-aided ontology-based systems such as the UMLS and D/P usually have three physical layers in the overall system architecture. The bottom layer is the database that contains the raw information arranged logically according to the consensus-certified ontological blueprint layout. On top of this layer is the middle layer semantic net, which is for machine execution and meticulously represents the logic of the ontological blueprint layout. The top layer is for the human users to interact with the ontology system and is the man-machine interface that fully captures the semantic net representation. The three layers should have-cross semantic transitivity, which means for any entities in any layer there are corresponding unambiguous representations in the other two layers. If a query is input by the user via the system interface (top layer), the query system would translate this into the request command understood by the semantic-net layer. The semantic-net layer then executes the command by invoking the retrieval algorithm (RA) to retrieve the requested data for the user. The three-layer conceptual architecture provides an effective ontological blueprint layout that is the prelude to a successful final robust ontology-based operational system.

Since the blueprint layout is to assist precise consensus-certification, its ontological details must be represented precisely and yet concisely enough for the certifiers to unambiguously understand them. Therefore, choosing an effective specification tool for the layout is prelude to success. Previous experience shows the tool should possess the following characteristics: (a) simple to use; (b) able to present details easily, clearly and unambiguously; (c) easy for the details in the layout to be translated into the corresponding semantic net; (d) contemporary in the sense that it migrates with time and technological advances to avoid sudden obsolescence; and (e) acts as a regulatory body that guides the evolution of the tool to meet new needs. For this reason, we have developed the Ontology Modelling Notation that was given in Sect. 3.4 and Appendix 1. Once the model in this Ontology Modelling Notation has been created, it is critiqued, evaluated and modified by the consensus certifiers to obtain an accurate and complete ontology model. This Model in the Ontology Modelling Notation is then transformed into a Design/Implementation Model that can be directly used for implementation of the Ontology.

The languages proposed by World Wide Web Consortium (W3C) for semantic-web purposes are good choices for the Design/Implementation Model, and they include:

(a) Extensible Markup Language (XML)—1st generation, namely XML, RDF and OWL family of metadata modeling tools proposed by the W3C, it is good at modeling semi-structured information but its capability to manipulate logical expressions is weak.
(b) Resource Description Framework (RDF)—2nd generation of the W3C metadata tools; it is more powerful than XML in handling logical expressions with weak logical transitivity (i.e. in terms of backtracking capability).
(c) Web Ontology Language (OWL)—3rd generation, compared to XML and RDF, with much stronger logic handling capability including backtracking and logical transitivity.

These are discussed in Chap. 3 and Appendix 2.

One of the biggest advantages of using W3C tools is that there are always supporting software packages in the field that can translate an ontological layout of a reasonable size into the corresponding semantic net representation and the supporting database automatically and correctly. The user needs to provide only the query interface to complete the final operational computer-aided ontology-based system.

Compared to XML, RDF and OWL, the Ontology Modelling Notation, given in Chap. 3, is also a unique modeling system that helps build relatively clear ontological layouts. It is simple to use and thus suitable for constructing the different modules of a sizeable ontological layout for consensus-certification purposes. There have been some attempts to use UML for Ontology Modelling. Unlike the W3C systems the problem with the UML representation [Cranefield01, Kogut02] is, however, that it lacks sufficient information for correct implementation. Figure 4.4 is used demonstrate this point. Here the logic of these UML parts in this ontological blueprint layout (e.g. logical points a and b) depend on the interpretation by the implementers (e.g. a can be AND, OR or EXCLUSIVE OR). This could lead to multiple representations of one concept and many incompatible implementations and eventual potential system failures. Multi-representations here mean that a single entity in the system has many different meanings leading to incongruent communication and understanding of the same concept. This is the source of ambiguity among different cognate systems resulting in erroneous operations. For practical purposes, therefore, a data-oriented system is preferred to the UML to allow the points a and b to converge to their true meaning with respect to the data set. In Fig. 4.4 the elements 0 and 5 are synonyms. The *retrieval algorithm* or RA_1 works by predicate logic; for example: (i) if "8" is true then "5" is true; (ii) if "9" is true then "6" is true; and (iii) if "5" and "6" are true then "3" is true (i.e. the logic for point "*b*" is a logical "AND" function). If for the same Fig. 4.4, another RA, namely RA_2, interprets point "*b*" as a logical OR (i.e. if "5" or "6" is true then "3" is true), then RA_1 and RA_2 are logically incompatible (i.e. $RA_1 \neq RA_2$). In our research, if one has to scrutinize the RA code in order to find out the exact meaning of "b", then the RA code has ***implicit*** semantics. Diagrammatically Fig. 4.4 does not differentiate the exact semantics between RA_1 and RA_2, and the two systems look similar superficially. Similarly, the implementation for the logical point "a" may vary from one system to another subject to the interpretations by the implementers, resulting in incompatible variants. Only when the predicates for different logical points in the variants are axiomatically defined and verified formally can we say whether they are actually clones.

In theory, any ontology correctly constructed from formal logic can be verified by the corresponding Petri net. To clarify this point, Fig. 4.5 is constructed as the formal Petri net representation of the "part of" hierarchy in Fig. 4.4, where logical point "a" (T2 should be fired) and "b" (T4 should be fired) have the OR and AND implementations respectively. In fact, this Petri-net construct can be used to simulate/check/specify the logical correctness of Fig. 4.4 [Kogut02, Dillon93]. The Petri net (PN) is bipartite and is made up of three sets of symbols arcs (A), transitions (T), and places (P) as follows: (a) PN = [P, T, A]; (b) P = [{1}, {2}, {3}, {4}, {5}, {6}, {7}, {8}, {9}, {10}]; and (c) T = [T1, T2, T3, T4, T5, T6, T7, T8, T9]. T1, T2 and T3 represent a logical OR operation and T4 the logical AND operation. Places {8} and {9} are initialized with two tokens (i.e. "*"). When a token is in a place then the place assumes the "true" state. T4 fires indeterminately as long as both places {5} and {6} have token(s). The transition firing is atomic,

Fig. 4.5 Formal Petri net
representation of Fig. 4.4

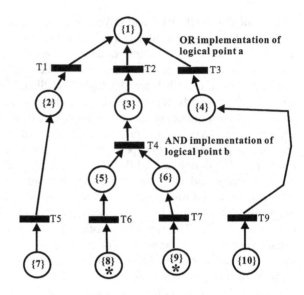

and this means that at anytime only one transition can fire even it takes zero time to complete. In Fig. 4.5 with the tokens in places {8} and {9}, the successive firing will generate the final token in place {3}, which represents the intermediate logical conclusion. In fact, the traversals starting from the places {8} and {9}, through the places {5}, {6} and {3}, finally for the token to reach place {1} represents a *"parsing"* process, which is the basic function of a semantic net. The traversals can be depicted clearly by the reachability graph in Fig. 4.6 in which the state vector changes with time when the transitions fire in an in-deterministic fashion. Every vector (e.g. M0) indicates the current state at the time, with a "1" to indicate the presence of a token—a "logically true" state. The leftmost bit position in the vector is for the place {1} and the rightmost for the place {10}.

Fig. 4.6 Reachability graph
for the Petri net in Fig. 4.5

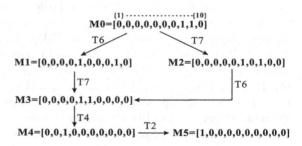

If we reverse the logical operations for the point "a" (i.e. to become logical AND) and "b" (i.e. to become logical OR), then the corresponding Petri net and its reachability graph will be very different. Therefore, logically speaking Fig. 4.5 differs from the Petri net with this reversal of the logical points *a* and *b* (i.e. "a" becomes "AND" and "b" becomes "OR") in another variant. Two variants, which are not clones, however, are still formal and axiomatic, but not logically compatible.

The walkthrough emphasizes the importance of choosing a good specification tool that can precisely represent the logical expressions clearly, formally and unambiguously. The most important of all is that these logical expressions can be visually checked easily. In this sense, an effective specification tool should have no hidden logical meanings that are subject to different interpretations by the implementers, as exemplified by the points *a* and b in Fig. 4.5.

Figure 4.7 is a 感冒 (flu) sub-ontology in an experimental web-based TCM system for clinical use. It was constructed by using XML as in Fig. 4.8.

In the domain of semantic web [Berners01], modeling languages such as XML, RDF, OWL and UML are commonly used for metadata modeling [Taniar06]. Therefore the realm of metadata modeling will be explored with some insight in the next section for ontology definitions.

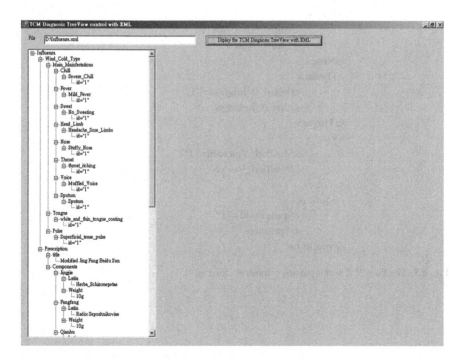

Fig. 4.7 Flu (病 = 感冒) sub-ontology attributes transcribed from medical canons

```
/* A <感冒> sub-ontology construct – pathological in nature */
<?xml version="1.0" encoding="Big5" ?>
<Influenza>
<Wind_Cold_Type>
<Main_Mainfestations>
    <Chill>
        <Severe_Chill>id="1"
        </Severe_Chill>
    </Chill>
    <Fever>
            <Mild_Fever>id="1"
            </Mild_Fever>
    </Fever>
    <Sweat>
            <No_Sweating>id="1"
            </No_Sweating>
    </Sweat>
    <Head_Limb>
            <Headache_Sore_Limbs>id="1"
            </Headache_Sore_Limbs>
    </Head_Limb>
            <Nose>
                    <Stuffy_Nose>id="1"
                    </Stuffy_Nose>
            </Nose>
            <Throat>
                    <throat_itching>id="1"
                    </throat_itching>
            </Throat>
            <Voice>
                    <Muffled_Voice>id="1"
                    </Muffled_Voice>
            </Voice>
            <Sputum>
                    <Sputum>id="1"
                    </Sputum>
            </Sputum>
```

Fig. 4.8 The flu <感冒> sub-ontology construct for Fig. 4.7

4.5 The Realm of Metadata Modeling

When an ontology blueprint layout is developed, there are some basic criteria that should be followed and they are as follows:

(a) The defined ontology should be accurate and easily altered (addition, deletion, and update modifications).
(b) The language/tool used should be a kind of de facto standard to reduce the chance of obsolescence.
(c) It should support semantic transitivity as well as easy logical extensions.

Metadata is the "data about data", which usually comes from a specific domain. Yet, the territory of metadata systems is very wide because there are many such systems, including the one supported by the World Web Consortium (W3C), namely XML, RDF, and OWL. These three metadata modelling languages can be nested at will among one another in a single model/document because they are cognate versions. *This characteristic is very useful for modelling because the three metadata systems can be nested for optimal document constructions* [W3Cc].

A metadata can be a simple content item or a construct of multiple content items. It facilitates understanding and management of data items as well as the associations among them. For example, it is often used to support locating and retrieving information. Metadata systems have existed for a long time in various forms; the table of contents (TOC) for a book is the one of the most common metadata used to describe the book's organization (e.g. authors, chapters, and publication date). In a library, the TOC (Table of Contents) metadata helps librarians organize the shelves to enable easy location of any book.

More sophisticated definitions of metadata arise out of new needs. For example, metadata may be regarded as structured and encoded data that describes the characteristics of information-bearing entities. The aim is to aid identification, discovery, assessment, and management of the described entities [ALA99]. For other applications, metadata is a set of optional structured descriptions that are publicly available to explicitly assist in locating objects [Bultermann04]. Therefore, it is reasonable to generalize metadata to a means to describe the structure, management, and usage of information in a domain.

Metadata usage covers a wide spectrum, and includes:

(a) Speeding up and enriching the search of web objects: This is typified by web browsers, P2P applications and file management software. Usually metadata improves the speed of file searches.
(b) Linking files: Documents can be converted into an electronic format that eases the storage in the document repository, such as Documentum; this facilitates the file retrieval process.
(c) Bridging semantic gaps, because the relationships between data items can be axiomatically specified: In this way it helps complex information retrieval operations. For example, if the search engine acquired the knowledge that "Aristotle" was a "Greek philosopher", users may provide a search query on

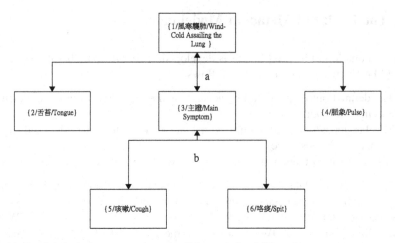

Fig. 4.9 Implicit logical representation—implicit semantics (bilingual)

"Greek philosopher" with a link to a Web page about "Aristotle", even if the exact term "Greek philosopher" never occurs in that page. This approach is generally called "Knowledge Representation", which is usually of special interest for applications in the areas of semantic web [Taniar06, Bultermann04; Berners01, ALA99] and artificial intelligence.

There are some strong arguments put forth in previous different publications (e.g. [JWong08a, JWong09d]) that the correct application of metadata systems would lead to logical correctness and completeness of a system design [IBM03]. This completeness applies to the functional aspects of the design itself. For example, if the implicit logic in the points *a* and *b* in the system shown in Fig. 4.9 is made explicit by appropriate metadata representation (e.g. RDF), then this system can be converted into the corresponding Petri net (e.g. Fig. 3.3 in Chap. 3). Through reachability analysis (e.g. Fig. 3.4 in Chap. 3), the logical correctness and completeness can be verified. If a metadata representation of the desired system of logical correctness and completeness can be converted into the final prototype in a single step, then it not only guarantees correct and smooth system operation but also eliminates the costs for debugging and maintenance. This is exactly what the new and innovative software engineering paradigm *Enterprise Ontology Driven Information System Development* (EOD-ISD [JWong08a]), described in Chap. 6, aims at.

4.6 Enterprise TCM Ontology Core

Ontology is a way to organized knowledge so that knowledge can be passed or exchanged in an unambiguous or formal manner. In the domain of philosophy, ontology deals with both facts and validity based on the pre-defined axioms.

Something is syllogistically correct if it is logical valid based on some of the axioms. Yet, validity does not mean truth or the time. Yet, in some applications, for example, clinical medicine, the emphasis is more on fact than validity. In commercial ontology constructs from which the managerial decision are drawn, facts are important because it determines profits or losses. Therefore, the ontological constructs for enterprises (i.e. enterprise ontology [JWong09c]) to gain the required benefits are normally based on facts. These facts should be presented in predefined forms, formats, nomenclature and terminology to facilitate unambiguous enterprise-wide communication and inter-operability. This formalism is the prelude to enterprise success nowadays because contemporary enterprises usually span over different continents and involve different people and language groups. Even people speak the same language (e.g. English), the same word may carry somewhat different meanings in addition to common semantics; that is, multi-representations. Some surveys multi-representations are the serious hurdle to software technology advancement in terms of cost and effectiveness. It is still the same for the percentage of software project failure nowadays as it was three decades ago, despite the frequent emergence of so called novel techniques and technologies [Osterweil08, Boehm08, Cheah07].

The success of computer-aided ontology-based enterprise systems depends on the following factors:

(i) Explicit specification of the ontological conceptualization: The drive is to ensure that the entities and their associations/relationships within the knowledge are formalized unambiguously to facilitate human understanding, interoperability and machine process [Gruber93a]. The World Wide Web Consortium (W3C) proposed to answer the unambiguous formalization part by knowledge annotation via metadata systems. As a result the W3C proposed the three "inter-nest-able" metadata system, namely, XML, RDF and OWL. Figure 4.9 shows part of the Nong's enterprise TCM onto-core, which is annotated with the three W3C metadata systems in an intertwined manner. This kind of knowledge annotation is 2-dimensional (2D) in nature even though it embeds a 3-dimensional (3D) hierarchical structure, which Guarino [Guarino95] called the subsumption hierarchy. This 2D annotation may suit humans who are used to textual reading, but it also leaves room to misunderstanding and imagination, for the 3-dimensional (3D) ambit is hard to visualize.

(ii) Logical machine operation: With respect to Guarino's concept [Guarino95], the machine works with the ontological knowledge by inference. Thus, it is logical to facilitate this inference or parsing by accentuating the subsumption hierarchy embedded in the ontology into a 3-D semantic net or document object model (DOM) tree. Structurally, the semantic net or DOM tree is made up of many semantic paths, and a parsing operation is to infer/draw the logical conclusion from the "complete logical path". For example, if the complete logical path is the following, where $\rightarrow$ indicates the hierarchical layer in descending order, $A \rightarrow B \rightarrow C \rightarrow D$, the possible inference consequences are: (i) for *Query*

```
<?xml version="1.0" encoding="big5" ?        /* Chinese only */>
<!DOCTYPE          rdf:RDF          [<!ENTITY          xsd
"http://www.w3.org/2001/XMLSchema#">]>
  <rdf:RDF
        xmlns:rdf="http://www.w3.org/1999/02/22-rdf-syntax-ns#"
        xmlns:rdfs="http://www.w3.org/2000/01/rdf-schema#"
        xmlns:xsd="http://www.w3.org/2001/XMLSchema#"
        xmlns:tcm="c:/testSchema#"
        xml:base="file:///./#">
  <tcm:病名 rdf:ID="感冒" />
  <tcm:證型 rdf:ID="風寒證">
        <rdfs:subClassOf rdf:resource="#感冒"/>
        <tcm:兼證 rdf:ID="風寒證兼證">口不渴或渴喜熱飲</tcm:兼
證>
        <tcm:舌苔 rdf:ID="風寒證舌苔">舌苔薄白</tcm:舌苔>
        <tcm:脈象 rdf:ID="風寒證脈象">脈象浮或兼緊</tcm:脈象>
  </tcm:證型>
  <tcm:主證 rdf:ID="風寒證主證">
        <rdfs:subClassOf rdf:resource="#風寒證"/>
  </tcm:主證>
  <tcm:衛表 rdf:ID="風寒證衛表">
        <rdfs:subClassOf rdf:resource="#風寒證主證"/>
        <tcm:怕冷 rdf:ID="風寒證怕冷">怕冷重</tcm:怕冷>
        <tcm:發熱 rdf:ID="風寒證發熱">發熱輕</tcm:發熱>
```

Fig. 4.10 An excerpt of the Nong's enterprise TCM onto-core

(A) $\Rightarrow$ B; (ii) for *Query*(A, B) $\Rightarrow$ C; (iii) for *Query*(A, B, C) $\Rightarrow$ D; (iv) for *Query*(A, C) $\Rightarrow$?/" *NoAnswer* "/" *undefined*". The left-most window in Fig. 4.10 is the semantic net for the partial ontology shown in Fig. 4.9.

(iii)   Syntactical operation: This is the query system where queries are constructed from the input parameters by the user. For example, *Query* (A, B) is constructed from the two user-specified parameters A and B. If the query system on top can construct all the logically correct queries from the given parameters, it basically abstracts the complete semantic net in the middle, which in its turn, abstracts the complete ontology at the bottom. If the cross-layer abstractions are perfect, then the cross-layer semantic transitivity exists. That is, if a logical entity is picked from a layer, its corresponding representations in the other two layers should surface in a consistent fashion. The right-most window of Fig. 4.10 abstracts the syntactical layer conceptually because the input/selected parameters are high-lighted in the semantic net. The middle-window abstracts the parsing mechanism (the parser software is only implied) and in this case the logical conclusion drawn by parser is "感冒" or flu of the = "風寒證" nature. In fact, the operation

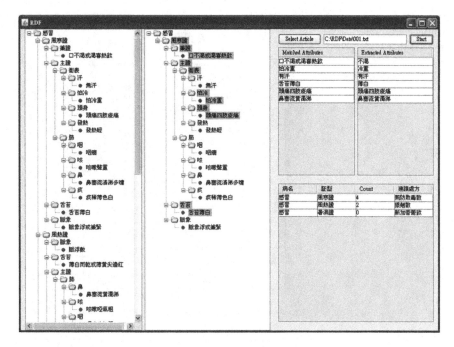

Fig. 4.11   Left-most window is the semantic net or DOM tree of Fig. 4.10

represented by screen capture in Fig. 4.11 is called *semantic transitivity visu-alization* (STV) and the tool to do this is the *semantic transitivity visualizer* or simple the STV tool [JWong09d].

4.7   Cross-Layer Onto-Core Semantic Transitivity (COST)

We would walk through the COST concept more clearly with the help of Figs. 4.12, 4.13 and 4.14.

Figure 4.12 is the result of when "Treeview" button was pressed with the selected "咳嗽" (cough) parameter. In the tree-view display the partial DOM tree that lists the herbs (i.e. 夏枯草—Spica Prunellae) in the left window for treating the symptom "咳嗽". The tree can be scrolled for scrutiny. The steps invoking the display are marked (circled). In effect, the user query in this case is *Query*{咳嗽}. The parsed result includes all the usable herbs that treat "咳嗽", as shown by the corresponding partial DOM tree. The parser is a mechanism that works on the semantic-net; it traces out the semantic path "夏枯草" (i.e. logical conclusion by inference) for the parameter "咳嗽". The corresponding herbs for treating "咳嗽" can be displayed in the textual form for simplicity. This is shown in Fig. 4.13 in which the steps for textual display invocation are marked. The textual display is

Fig. 4.12 DOM tree or
semantic net display for the
query (咳嗽)

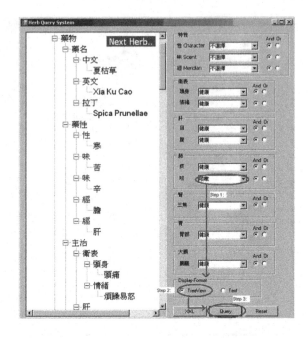

Fig. 4.13 Text display for the
herbs that treat "咳嗽"

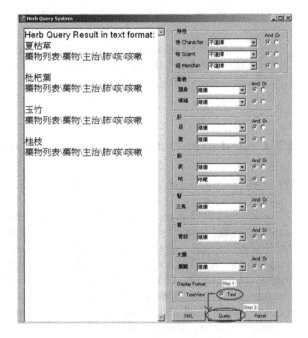

Fig. 4.14 Semantic-transitive cross-referencing display

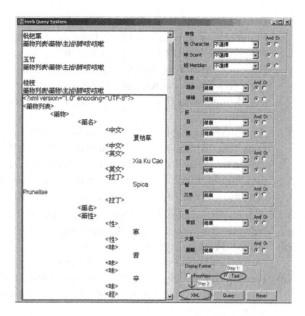

basically extracted from the annotated ontological layer, which is open to any kind of language (e.g. English, Chinese, etc.).

Figure 4.14 is the screen capture of the partial EHS, which is annotated in XML. This partial XML code shown corresponds to the partial DOM tree for parsing the query, *Query*{咳嗽}. In the COST concept, the learner is free to choose how to cross-reference the three ontological layers: (i) syntactical on the top; (ii) semantic net or DOM tree in the middle; and (iii) ontological annotation at the bottom. Cross-referencing is useful for anybody, TCM expert or not, to visualize and check if the parser, which is otherwise invisible, functions logically, anywhere and anytime.

4.8 COST Check Anytime and Anywhere

Cross-layer onto-core semantic transitivity (COST) checking should be part of the TCM telemedicine framework; formally it is called semantic transitivity visualization (STV). In this case, the GUI has the following blocks that each represents and icon in the iconic specification:

(a) Patient icon/block: This block allows the user to key-in any patient information including family medical history for recording purposes (i.e. case building).

(b) Diagnosis icon/block: It has several small windows including: (i) Main Symptom—the main complaint from the patient (in this case "loath ambient temperature"); (ii) Other Symptom—the main syndrome with respect to the complaint; (iii) Tongue—tongue diagnosis which is a main diagnostic procedure; (iv) Pulse—another main diagnostic procedure; and (v) Diagnosis—the keyed-in answers (by the user/physician) from the patient (real/simulated) are echoed.

(c) Illness: The possible diagnoses drawn by the parser from the keyed-in symptoms. The likelihood of these diagnoses with respect to the input symptoms is ranked by the overall relevance index (RI) values. In the enterprise ontology, all the symptoms with respect to different illnesses are ranked during the last round of consensus certification. Thus, the "overall" RI value for a set of symptoms with respect to an illness can be conceptualized by $RI_j = \sum_{i=1}^{n} s_i^j$, where i and j indicates the symptom and the illness respectively.

(d) Herbal: For the set of input symptoms $\{s_i | i = 1, 2, \ldots, n\}$, all the usable herbs are ranked by the corresponding RI vales.

(e) Prescription: It helps the physician/learner/user to select the supposedly most suitable herbs (with the highest RI values) for creating the prescription for treating the patient (Fig. 4.15).

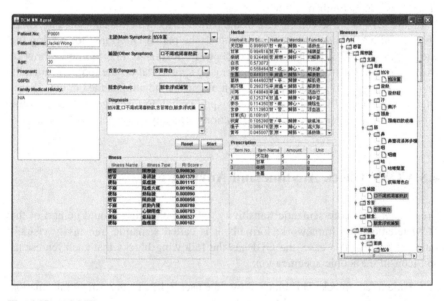

Fig. 4.15 A COST screen capture

4.9 Recapitulation

In the next chapter, we will show examples of how a successful proprietary TCM ontology of industrial standard can be used for Ontology Based System generation.

References

[ALA99] American Library Association: Task Force on Metadata Summary Report, June 1999

[Berners01] Berners-Lee, T., James, H., Ora, L.: The semantic web, scientific American magazine, 17 May 2001

[Bultermann04] Bultermann, DCA.: Is it time for a moratorium on metadata? IEEE MultiMedia **11**(4), 10–17 (2004) (Oct–Dec)

[Cranefield01] Cranefield, S., Haustein, S., Purvis, M.: UML-based ontology modelling for software agents. In: Proceedings of the 5th international conference on autonomous agents, Montreal, Canada, 28 May–1 June 2001

[Dillon93] Dillon, T.S.: Object Oriented Conceptual Modeling, Prentice Hall, 1993

[Dillon14] Dillon, T.S., Chang, E.J., Rahayu, W.: Object Oriented Conceptual Modelling and Design. CRL Publishing Ltd., UK (2014)

[Gruber93a] Gruber, T.R.: A translation approach to portable ontology specification. Knowl. Acquis. **5**(2), 199–220 (1993)

[Guarino95] Guarino, N., Giaretta, P.: Ontologies and knowledge bases: towards a terminological clarification. Towards Very Large Knowl. Bases Knowl. Build. Knowl. Sharing, 25–32 (1995)

[IBM03] IBM and Sandpiper Software Incorporated, Ontology definition meta-model, http://www.omg.org/docs/ad/05-8-01.pdf (2003). Accessed 14 December 2008

[Kogut02] Kogut, P., Cranefield, S., Hart, L., Dutra, M., Baclawski, K., Kokar, M., Smith, J.: UML for ontology development. Knowl. Eng. Rev. **17**(1), 61–64 (2002). Journal Special Issue on Ontologies in Agent Systems

[JWong08c] Plenary keynote—Tele-medicine: Application to Traditional Chinese Medicine (TCM), IEEE-DEST2008, Phitsanulok, Thailand, 25–29 Feb 2008

[Taniar06] Taniar, D., Rahayu, J. (ed.): Web Semantics and Ontology. Idea Group Incorporated (2006)

[UMLS] UMLS http://umls.nlm.nih.gov/

[W3Ca] W3C: Ontology Definition MetaModel (2005). http://www.omg.org/docs/ad/05-08-01.pdf#search='Ontology%20Definition%20Metamodel

[W3Cb] W3C: Web Service Architecture (Working Paper). http://www.w3.org/TR/ws-arch/

[W3Cc] W3C Web site. http://www.w3.org/

[WHO07] WHO: International Standard Terminologies on Traditional Medicine in the Western Pacific Region. World Health Organization (2007). ISBN 978-92-9061-248-7

[JWong08a] Wong, J.H.K., Dillon, T.S., Wong, A.K.Y., Lin, W.W.K.: Text mining for real-time ontology evolution. In: Data Mining for Business Applications, pp. 143–150. Springer, Berlin (2008), ISBN: 978-0-387-79419-8

[JWong09a]   Wong, J.H.K., Wong, A.K.Y., Lin W.W.K., Dillon, T.S.: A novel approach to achieve real-time TCM (Traditional Chinese Medicine) telemedicine through the use of ontology and clinical intelligence discovery. Int. J. Comput. Syst. Sci. Eng. (CSSE) **24**(4), 219–240 (2009)

[JWong09c]   Wong, J.H.K., Lin, W.W.K., Wong, A.K.Y., Dillon, T.S.: TCM (Traditional Chinese Medicine) telemedicine with enterprise ontology support—a form of consensus-certified collective human intelligence. In: Proceedings of the International Conference on Industrial Technology (ICIT), Monash University, Victoria, Australia, 10–13 Feb 2009

[JWong09d]   Wong, J.H.K.: Ph.D. Thesis: Web-based Data Mining and Discovery of Useful Herbal Ingredients (***WD²UHI***). Department of Computing, Hong Kong Polytechnic University (2009)

Chapter 5
Ontology Driven System Generation and Remote Installation

5.1 Introduction

The Nong's mobile clinics (MC) provide a successful example of telemedicine in the TCM domain. The "diagnosis/prescription (D/P)" system that supports the MC has been treating hundreds patients in the Hong Kong SAR since its deployment four year ago. The D/P success can be attributed to the following innovations:

- (i)   enterprise ontology core (in this case it is the TCM ontology core or onto-core).
- (ii) cross-layer onto-core semantic transitivity (COST).
- (iii) error-free system customization based on the meta-interface (MI) concept.
- (iv) automatic remote web-based installation.
- (v)   "living" onto-core to support on-line evolution.
- (vi) knowledge and experience re-absorption.
- (vii) COST check anytime, anywhere and by another body with some TCM knowledge.

In the last chapter we considered: (i) the TCM ontology core or onto-core; and (ii) cross-layer onto-core semantic transitivity. In this chapter, we will discuss: (iii) error-free system customization based on the meta-interface (MI) concept through the use of the TCM Onto Core and the enterprise Icon Library to carry out automated Information System generation for use at a 'local site'; and (iv) automatic remote web-based installation at a 'local site'.

5.2 The Mobile-Clinic Experience Unveils the Importance of Ontological Adherence

Figure 5.1 shows a network of collaborating D/P systems in a Nong's MC setup. Every mobile clinic system or MC is a self-contained atomic clinic/unit, which has the several essential elements: (i) on-board physician(s); (ii) on-board pharmacy; (iii) paramedic;

© Springer-Verlag Berlin Heidelberg 2015   99
A.K.Y. Wong et al., *Semantically Based Clinical TCM Telemedicine Systems*,
Studies in Computational Intelligence 587, DOI 10.1007/978-3-662-46024-5_5

(iv) patient registration; (v) smart space support that connects the MC to the PCI (pervasive computing infrastructure); and (vi) central management and support. Although every MC is conceptually self-sufficient under normal circumstances, external help is still needed under various situations; for example, second diagnostic opinions, toxicity control, patient record retrieval, and on-line inventory update of drugs. To ensure that all the MC units are communicating correctly, a standard vocabulary is needed to avoid ambiguity. In this light, ontological adherence is an advantage. Figure 5.1 illustrates how different MC variants, which are generated by the MI concept, are still able to communicate because every variant has a subset of the overall enterprise vocabulary {V}. In a high-level sense {V} abstracts the master enterprise TCM onto-core, from which the other local TCM onto-cores are customized by the EOD-ISD mechanism (a realization of the MI concept).

Figure 5.2 shows the MI concept, which is realized as the EOD-ISD mechanism. The three basic components in the EOD-ISD framework are as follows:

(a) Master TCM onto-core: This ontology defines the ambit of operation of the enterprise owner. It has an explicit subsumption hierarchy, namely, the semantic net or DOM tree.
(b) Standard vocabulary {V}: The enterprise that owns the master TCM onto-core above would maintain a standard vocabulary {V} to abstract the onto-core. In reality {V} is the onto-core with an implicit subsumption hierarchy.
(c) Enterprise icon library (IL): It is the repertoire of system building experience. Every icon is basically a semantic path in the semantic net. If $A \rightarrow B \rightarrow C$ is a semantic path, where $\rightarrow$ means "implying", then three possible icons can be defined, namely: $A \rightarrow B$, $B \rightarrow C$, and $A \rightarrow B \rightarrow C$.

The MI paradigm is a novel software engineering approach called semantic or iconic programming. The user needs to formulate only the iconic specification, which is made up of the icons selected from the Enterprise Icon Library (IL). With the iconic specification as the input, the EOD-ISD mechanism automatically generates the target ontology-based system with a 3-layer architecture. The iconic

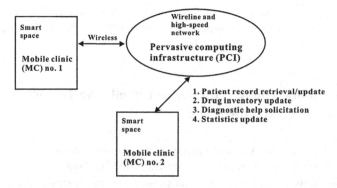

Fig. 5.1 Nong's MC-based telemedicine perspective

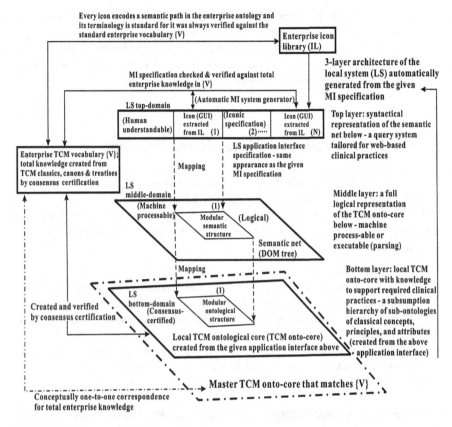

Fig. 5.2 MI concept—EOD-ISD mechanism

specification normally looks the same as the GUI of the target system generated by the EOD-ISD mechanism. With the same iconic specification, the same target systems (or clones) would be repeatedly generated by the EOD-ISD mechanism. Different iconic specifications would produce different cognate target systems or variants because the local TCM onto-core modules of these systems are basically derivatives of the same master TCM onto-core. All the clones and variants can communicate among themselves to a varying degree because their "local vocabulary" is a subset of {V}. This shows the importance of ontological adherence because users of all the variants can communicate unambiguously due to {V}.

Figure 5.2 also shows the essence of the following elements:

(a) Iconic specification: It is for human understanding and manipulation.

(b) GUI of the target system: From the iconic specification the EOD-ISD mechanism generates the target system of a 3-layer architecture: (i) GUI—as the top (1st) syntactical layer for query formation, for example $Query(x_1, x_2)$ where (x_1, x_2) is the set of input parameters/attributes; (ii) "semantic net + parser"—as the middle (2nd) layer for machine understanding and processing where the parser infers the semantic net for a logical conclusion for the input $Query(x_1, x_2)$; and (iii) local onto-core that defines the ambit of operation for the local system, and this ambit is implicitly contained in the iconic specification. The GUI completely hides the 3-layer system architecture.

5.3 Provision of Standard Diagnosis and Prescription

The diagnosis/prescription (D/P) system variant shown in Fig. 5.3 was generated from the given iconic specification by the EOD-ISD mechanism.

The GUI screen captured is shown in Fig. 5.3. In this case, the GUI has the following blocks that each represents an icon in the iconic specification explained more fully in Chap. 4:

(a) Patient icon/block.
(b) Diagnosis icon/block: It has several small windows including: (i) Main Symptom; (ii) Other Symptoms; (iii) Tongue; (iv) Pulse; and (v) Diagnosis—the keyed-in answers (by the user/physician) from the patient (real/simulated) are echoed.
(c) Illness: The possible diagnoses drawn by the parser from the keyed-in symptoms, ranked by the overall RI (relevance index) values.

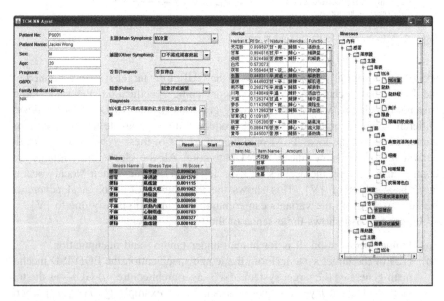

Fig. 5.3 A COST screen capture

(d) Herbal: The usable herbs ranked by the corresponding RI vales.
(e) Prescription: It helps the physician/learner/user to select the most suitable
     herbs (with the highest RI values) for creating the prescription for treating the
     patient.

The iconic specification is comprised of all the icons in the icon library shown in
Fig. 5.4. The user can create the iconic specification by moving the icons (i.e.
"add") one by one to the right box and pressing "Generate" to automate the D/P
system generation process. In fact, the "Add All" and "Generate" sequence had
generated the D/P system variant shown in Fig. 5.3.

Figure 5.3 is just the GUI of the 3-layer ontology-based system. It has shown the
middle semantic net partially in the rightmost box. The semantic net is the subsumption hierarchy if the local TCM onto-core extracted/customized from the
master Nong's TCM onto-core in this case. The local TCM onto-core complete
define the ambit of D/P operation by the local D/P system. In effect, it is the local
system vocabulary {V}. Since the operation of the system in Fig. 5.3 is key-in
based, the user/physician selects the symptoms by clicking the different boxes
selectively. All the keyed-in symptoms are standard and echoed in the "Diagnosis"
box to acknowledge the user inputs. If the "Start" button is pushed, GUI/syntactical
layer will build the corresponding query to be parsed by the middle layer (Fig. 5.5).
That is, the parser infers and draws the logical conclusion from the semantic net for
the input query. Since every icon in the iconic specification is a semantic path, all

Fig. 5.4 Icon library and
iconic specification

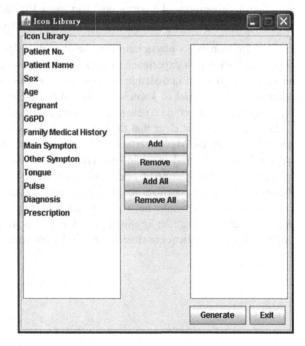

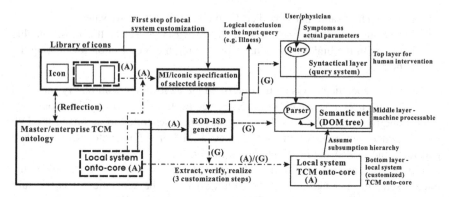

Fig. 5.5 Iconic MI customization flow with enterprise ontology support

the icons in the specification together form the overall semantic net in the middle layer. And, in this sense there should be a logical conclusion for every query, which itself a semantic path.

In Fig. 5.3 the parser infers the corresponding answers for the input query, and these answers include:

(a) Relevant illnesses: The relevancies of these illnesses are indicated by the RI (relevance index) scores; the one with the highest RI score is the most likely.
(b) Relevant ingredient for treatments: All the possible ingredients for treatment are ranked and listed. Then, the physician based on his own experience and the current geographical environment can make the suitable prescription utilizing the information provided in the ranked list of possible ingredients.

The decision by a physician to make the most appropriate prescription with respect to his/her past experience as well as the current geographical environment is an important piece of knowledge to others when shared with them. In light of TCM telemedicine, this kind of knowledge should be re-absorbed into enterprise ontology to enrich the latter via a new of consensus certification, as explained in Chap. 6.

From Fig. 5.3 it is clear that the ontology-based telemedicine system generated automatically by the Meta Interface (MI) approach is a very effective way to provide standard diagnosis and prescription. This is achieved because: (a) the local D/P system is completed defined by its iconic specification; (b) with iconic specification the MI mechanism customizes the ontology-based system of three layers: (i) top GUI layer; (ii) middle "semantic net + parser" layer; and (iii) bottom ontology layer with proper annotations; (c) the key-in approach enforces unambiguous query constructions; and (d) the logical conclusions drawn by the parser are ranked.

5.4 Error-Free System Customization
   by the Meta-Interface (MI) Concept

The MI approach supported by automatic code generation and remote system installation for customizing clinical telemedicine systems (e.g. the Nong's mobile-clinic D/P system) is also known as *the enterprise ontology driven information system development* (EOD-ISD) paradigm. Typically, this paradigm is supported by the given enterprise ontology in mind (e.g. Nong's TCM onto-core) [Uschold07]. It is superior to the traditional software engineering methodology represented by the Waterfall model, which usually starts with the user/functional specification and may involve the fast prototyping process that allows user input and participation in different development phases. From the user functional specification, the design specification is derived, verified and implemented. Effective change control can be achieved in various ways; such as by monitoring the entity-relationships so that variables and functions would not be inadvertently modified, causing errors in system operation. Yet, the semantics of the program modules are not explicit, making their reusability and debugging difficult. This is particular so if the software is for distributed processing because traditional debugging tools designed for sequential processing are not applicable.

Figure 5.5 concisely depicts the essence of the MI paradigm as follows:

(a) Library of icons: The icons can be defined by anyone to be used by others. Every icon reflects a semantic path in the master/enterprise ontology (TCM onto-core in this case as an example).

(b) MI/iconic specification: It is made up of selected icons from the library of icons. In this case the iconic specification of selected icons is represented by (A). In reality (A) is a reflection of the ontological portion in the enterprise ontology, and this portion is going to be the "local system onto-core" of the customized/target system.

(c) EOD-ISD generator: It extracts portion (A) from the enterprise ontology according to the iconic specification, which is a reflection of (A). The generator automatically generates [i.e. (G)] the "query system (syntactical layer on top)", the "semantic net/DOM tree (middle layer)", and the "local system onto-core (bottom layer)". To complete the customization process, the generator has to include the following "standard modules" to be supplied by the enterprise (e.g. Nong's): (i) the parser software; and (ii) the library of query generation algorithms. Therefore, for the top layer the EOD-ISD generates not only the graphical user interface (GUI) but includes the "standard library of algorithms". For the middle layer, the standard parser software is included as part of the automatic system generation process. The system generation process (G) may be summarized by three steps: extract (from the master/enterprise ontology), verify (if the extraction is correct), and realize (the 3-layer architecture: top syntactical layer; middle logical semantic net; and the bottom onto-core). Every customized target system is a variant of the "master" system supported by the complete enterprise ontology. The ambit of functionality of every variant is dictated by the local onto-core.

The GUI of any customized system looks exactly the same as its iconic specification, and it hides the details in the 3-layer architecture. Figure 5.6 is an example, and the GUI in this case was customized from a user-provided iconic specification employing the same ten selected icons namely:

(a) **Section (I)—The bar of control icons**.
(b) **Section (II)**—Patient registration number (or diagnostic Identifier) (i.e. MX6060303001) waiting for treatment and the important fields to be filled later: (i) patient's complaint ("主訴"); and ii) diagnosis ("診斷"): illness/type ("病"/"証"), and the treatment principle ("治則治法").
(c) **Section (III)**—Symptoms ("現病史") obtained by a standard TCM diagnostic procedure that has been crystallized from eons of clinical experience.

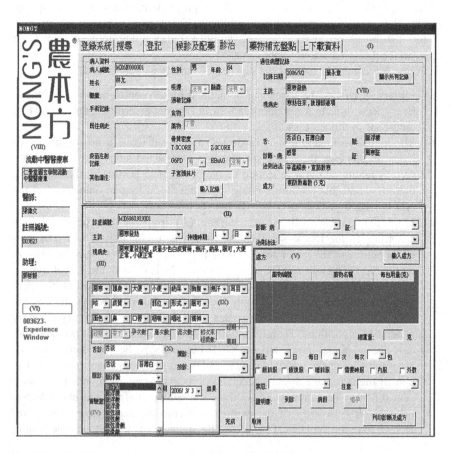

Fig. 5.6 D/P GUI generated from the given MI by EOD-ISD

Table 5.1 A traditional "望, 聞, 問, 切" diagnosis example (manual conclusion)

Look (望)	Listen&smell (聞)	Question (問)	Pulse-diagnosis (切)	Illness concluded
Pale face	Cough, bad breath	Headache, fever, loathe cold ambience conditions (惡寒/怕冷)	Taut and fast	Influenza (感冒)

(d) **Section (IV)—Pulse diagnosis ("脈診").**

(e) **Section (V)**—Prescription(s) ("處方") for the diagnosis filled in section (II); printing the final prescription and dispensing it directly in the MC.

(f) **Section (VI)**—Experience window (repository) entrance of the logon TCM physician with unique official medical practice registration number (e.g. 003623 as shown).

(g) **Section (IX)**—Specific questions (e.g. Do you loathe cold ambience conditions ("惡寒/怕冷")?), and general physical inspection (e.g. complexion ("面色")—pale, red or dark).

(h) **Section (X)—Tongue diagnosis ("舌診") (e.g. texture and coating color).**

In Fig. 5.6, the "Symptoms (現病史)" window echoes the symptoms obtained from the patient by the normal four-step diagnostic procedure: Look (望), Listen&Smell (聞), Question (問), and Pulse-diagnosis (切). Table 5.1 shows an example of how these four steps would be applied by the physician to reach a diagnostic conclusion in the traditional and manual way; in this case Influenza (感冒) is concluded. With the D/P interface a physician follows the same four steps, but in a "key-in", computer-aided fashion. The "key-in" D/P operation is standard and potentially allows the D/P results to be used as immediate feedback to enrich the local TCM onto-core. This is possible because all the TCM terms in the "select & key-in procedure" are standard in the enterprise ontology or vocabulary and thus the local system ontology customized by the EOD-ISD process. All the translations of Chinese terms into English in the master enterprise TCM onto-core are based on the World Health Organization (WHO) TCM standard [WHO07]. The master TCM onto-core may be annotated by various metadata systems. For example, the master Nong's TCM onto-core is annotated by the three inter-nest-able W3C metadata systems, namely XML, RDF, and OWL (e.g. Fig. 4.10 in Chap. 4).

Figure 5.7 is the English GUI generated from an iconic specification, which indicated the same iconic requirements as Fig. 5.6. In fact, the EOD-ISD approach is multilingual and therefore suits TCM practitioners across the globe.

The EOD-ISD is a new paradigm that takes advantage of intrinsic explicit semantics expressed in the enterprise ontology. The success of the Nong's D/P telemedicine system is an evidence of the EOD-ISD effectiveness. The D/P system development process differentiates three conceptual levels of ontological constructs: (i) the global ontology; (ii) the local enterprise ontology core (onto-core); and (iii) the local system onto-core. In this light, the details of the three conceptual levels for clinical TCM practice are as follows:

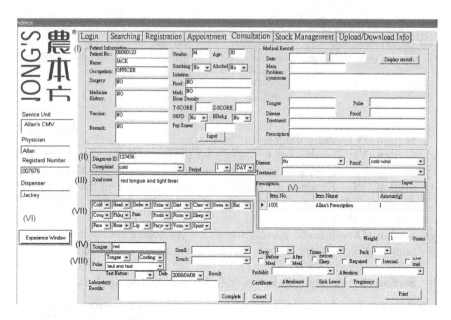

Fig. 5.7 GUI and diagnosis capture of the extant D/P (English version)

(a) Global TCM ontology: This includes knowledge from all the relevant TCM classics, medical theories (syllogistic—logically valid but may not have been verified yet), case histories, and treatises. It is an explicit conceptualization of concepts, entities, and their associations [Gruber93a], and this conceptualization may be organized into the corresponding subsumption hierarchy of sub-ontology constructs [Guarino95].

(b) Local TCM enterprise ontology (or simply enterprise ontology): This is a subset of the global TCM ontology extracted with a specific clinical purpose in mind. For example, the Nong's TCM onto-core is an extraction for clinical telemedicine deployment and practice. Therefore, the Nong's vocabulary reflects only clinical facts and no syllogistic assumptions.

Local Mobile Clinic (MC) D/P system TCM onto-core: It is customized directly from the Nong's proprietary or "master" TCM onto-core for the meta-interface (MI) specification given; thus it is a subset of the master TCM onto-core. The customization of a D/P system is automatic and the first step is to create the MI specification by selecting desired icons from the Nong's master icon library. Therefore, the local TCM onto-cores for all the MC systems customized for a particular client would be the same, but would differ from those of other clients. Neither the Nong's master TCM onto-core nor the local MC D/P system TCM onto-cores evolve automatically. In their present form, they all risk the danger becoming stagnated with only ancient TCM knowledge derived from old classics, treatises, and case histories. The proposal of the novel automatic semantic aliasing and text mining (ASA&TM) approach will remove this stagnation danger.

5.5 Automatic Remote Web-Based Installation

Automatic web-based installation is an important feature of the proprietary Nong's TCM telemedicine infrastructure [Lin08]. Any Nong's D/P (diagnosis/prescription) system invariant customized for a subscriber would be installed remotely anytime and anywhere over the Internet. The installation process involves two basic steps as follows:

(a) Nong's gives the subscriber the license/permission to download the D/P system into his pre-created home page.
(b) The customized D/P system is packed into a single package (e.g. as a "*.msi file*" in the Microsoft Visual Studio (MS-VS) environment), which contains many executable (.exe) files.

There are many ways that the Nong's would support automatic remote web-based D/P system installation, and the MS-VS (Microsoft Visual Studio) approach is a convenient approach, consisting of the following steps:

(a) Creating the subscriber's D/P system package: The package of code and data basically assumes the 3-layer architecture shown in Fig. 5.2; namely:

  • The top syntactical layer: This is the GUI and query system for the user to interact with the rest of the system; this layer basically represents human understanding of the ontological contents.
  • The middle semantic net: The parsing mechanism infers the logical conclusion from the semantic net for the input query. The semantic net of DOM tree should abstract the ontological contents perfectly.
  • The bottom ontology: It defines the ambit of the system functionality in a formal and classical sense.

  The screen capture to show this point is displayed by Fig. 5.8.
(b) Add files into the package: Since the files in a D/P package are multimedia in nature, the software engineer on the provider side (i.e. Nong's in this case) has to add relevant files selectively into the target D/P system package. Both screen captures in Figs. 5.9 and 5.10 illustrate this point.
(c) Format the D/P system package: This can be achieved by using the MS Installer as shown by Fig. 5.11. The screen capture in Fig. 5.12 shows that the MS Installer has built the target D/P system package successfully.
(d) Create the *named folder* for the target D/P system: This invokes remote installation. The *named folder* that contains the target D/P system in this case is called the "*Mobile Medicine Package Setup*".
(e) Remote installation: The client/subscriber, who has got the permission/license, can log-in the assigned *named folder* by "double-clicking" it to invoke/start the local installation at the client site. This involves two basic steps conceptually: (a) download the package, and (b) install the package locally. A successful remote installation invocation is indicated by the message "*Welcome to 'Mobile Medicine Package Setup*'" by *Setup Wizard* (Fig. 5.13). Then, the subscriber should press the "*Next*" button to start installing the D/P package in

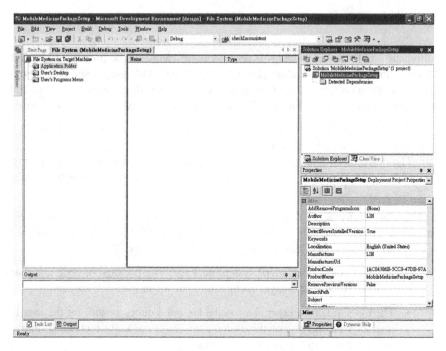

Fig. 5.8 Step 1—creating a subscriber's D/P package by visual studio (VS)

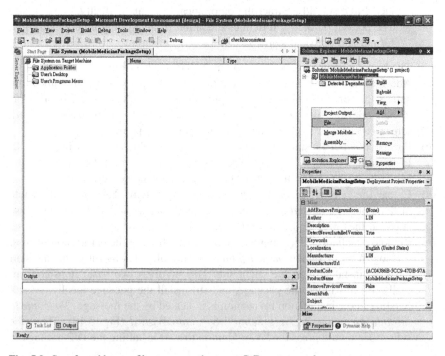

Fig. 5.9 Step 2—add more files to create the target D/P system package

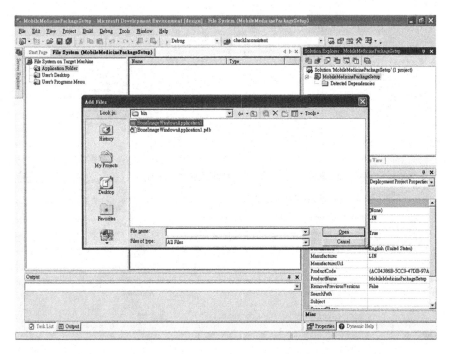

Fig. 5.10 Step 3—add more files to create the target D/P system package by VS

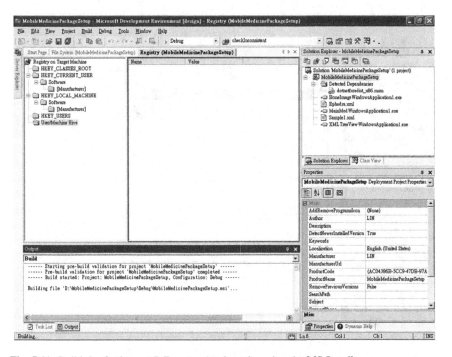

Fig. 5.11 Build the final target D/P system package by using the MS Installer

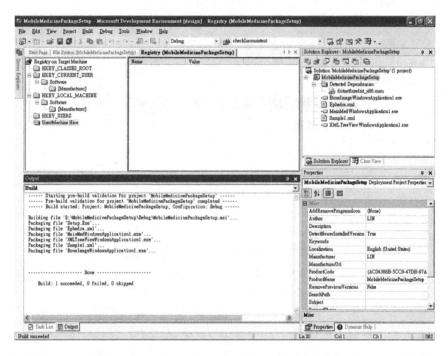

Fig. 5.12 Target D/P system package built successfully (ready for web transfer)

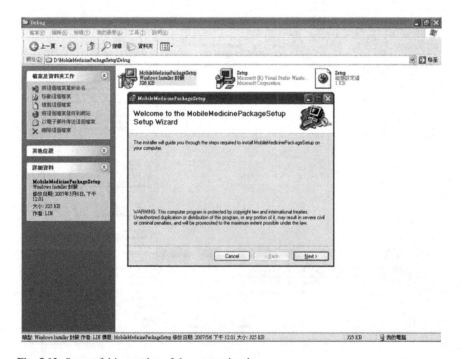

Fig. 5.13 Successful invocation of the setup wizard

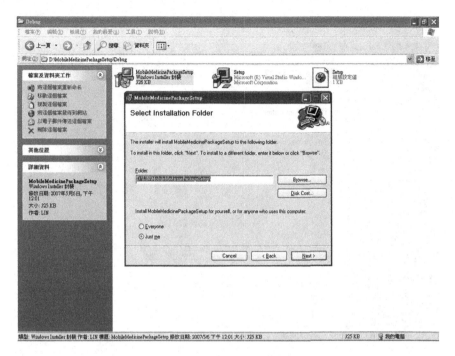

Fig. 5.14 D/P package will be installed into the "N/H" folder (client specified)

"named/home (N/H)" folder (Fig. 5.14), which is confirmed by the MS
Installer (Fig. 5.15). The Installer continues to indicate that the installation is
still in progress (Fig. 5.16). The successful installation of the local D/P system
was finally confirmed (Fig. 5.17), and all the related files in the home folder
(.exe and data) are shown in Fig. 5.18. All the installed items of the local D/P
system can be viewed by using the MS Window's Control Panel (Fig. 5.19).

5.6   Recapitulation

In this chapter, we explained the Enterprise Ontology Driven Information System
Development approach that automatically generates the "local software system and
associated sub ontology" that is utilized at a "local site". In that way, it can be
ensured that the "local sub ontology" is coherent with the Master Onto Core creating semantic interoperability. In addition we also explained how the "local
software system generated" can be remotely installed at a site remote from the
Master Onto Core Server. In the next chapter, we will consider the evolution of the
Master Onto Core, as new knowledge is extracted and consensus certified from new
cases that are being accumulated.

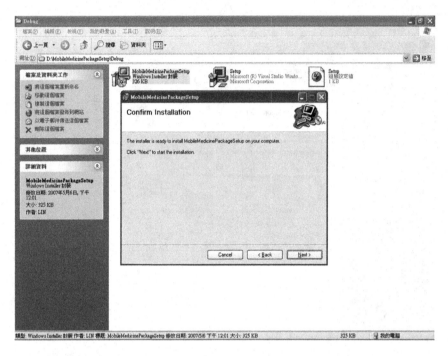

Fig. 5.15 MS installer confirms the start of the "N/H" D/P system installation

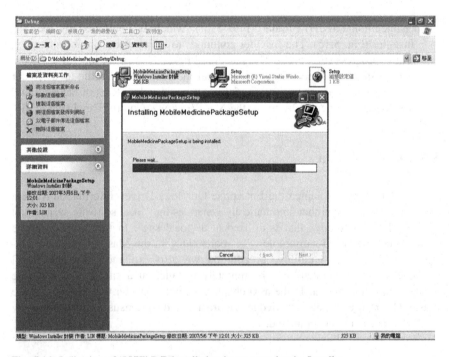

Fig. 5.16 Indication of "N/H" D/P installation in progress by the Installer

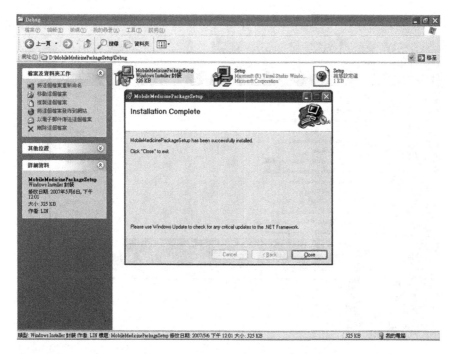

Fig. 5.17 D/P system "N/H" installation success indicated

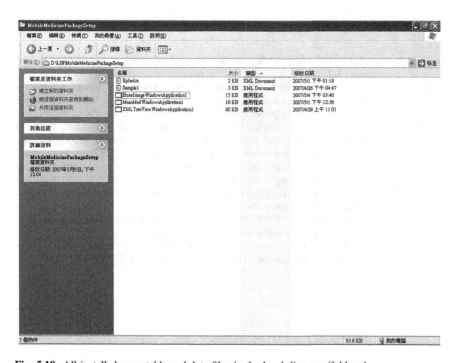

Fig. 5.18 All installed executable and data files in the local directory/folder show

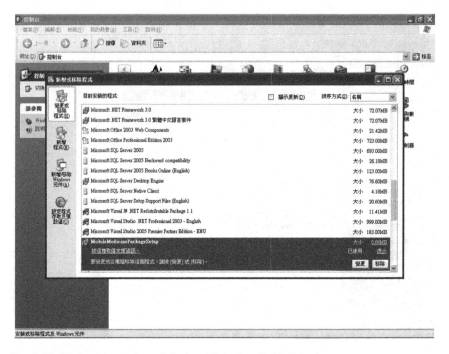

Fig. 5.19 Window's control panel displays all the installed D/P items

References

[Gruber93a]   Gruber, T.R.: A translation approach to portable ontology specification. Knowl. Acquis. **5**(2), 199–220 (1993)

[Guarino95]   Guarino, N., Giaretta, P.: Ontologies and knowledge bases: towards a terminological clarification. Towards Very Large Knowledge Bases: Knowledge Building and Knowledge Sharing, IOS Press, Amsterdam, pp. 25–32 (1995)

[Lin08]   Lin, W.W.K., Wong, J.H.K., Wong, A.K.Y.: Applying dynamic buffer tuning to help pervasive medical consultation succeed. In: Proceedings of the 1st International Workshop on Pervasive Digital Healthcare (PerCare), Proceedings of the 6th Annual IEEE International Conference on Pervasive Computing and Communications. Hong Kong, pp. 675–67917–21 Mar 2008

[Uschold07]   Uschold, M., King, M., Moralee, S., Zorgios, Y.: The Enterprise Entology, Artificial Intelligence Applications Institute. University of Edinburgh, UK. http://citesee.ist.psu.edu/cache/papers/cs/11430/ftp:zSzzSzftp.aiai.ed..ac.ukzSzpubzSzdocumentszSz1998zSz98-ker-ent-ontology.pdf/uschold95enterprise.pdf (2007)

[WHO07]   WHO: International Standard Terminologies on Traditional Medicine in the Western Pacific Region, World Health Organization (2007). ISBN 978-92-9061-248-7

Chapter 6
Ontology Evolution and the Living TCM Ontology

6.1 Introduction

As mentioned in Chap. 5, the success of this diagnosis/prescription (D/P) system can be attributed to the following innovations:

 (i) enterprise ontology core (in this case it is the TCM ontology core or onto-core)
 (ii) cross-layer onto-core semantic transitivity (COST)
 (iii) error-free system customization based on the meta-interface (MI) concept
 (iv) automatic remote web-based installation
 (v) "living" onto-core to support on-line evolution
 (vi) knowledge and experience re-absorption
 (vii) COST check anytime, anywhere and by another body with some TCM knowledge

In the Chap. 4, we considered (i) the TCM ontology core or onto-core and (ii) cross-layer onto-core semantic transitivity. In Chap. 6, this was followed by a discussion of (iii) error-free system customization based on the meta-interface (MI) concept to carry out automated Information System generation for use at a 'local site' (iv) automatic remote web-based installation at a 'local site'. In this chapter, we address (v) "living" onto-core to support on-line evolution and (vi) knowledge and experience re-absorption.

The need for evolution arises from a variety of sources including:

- Scientific advances leading to better understanding of the domain
- New Diagnostic techniques that become available including the use of ultra-sound and pathology tests
- New Disease types that have not been previously encountered. Examples of this include the SARS outbreak and HIV
- New treatments or prescriptions that are being used successfully by some clinical practitioners. In TCM, this is a very important source of new knowledge
- New environmental conditions

© Springer-Verlag Berlin Heidelberg 2015
A.K.Y. Wong et al., *Semantically Based Clinical TCM Telemedicine Systems*,
Studies in Computational Intelligence 587, DOI 10.1007/978-3-662-46024-5_6

Ontology Evolution [Stojanovic02, Khattak09, JWong09d] involves the timely but accurate adaptation of the Ontology to reflect new knowledge that has been properly certified by a team of experts.

There are several aspects to this Ontology evolution and they include:

(a) Identification of possible new knowledge
(b) Determination potential representation within the existing Master Onto Core
(c) Consensus certification of the potential representation by a team of domain experts
(d) Enhancing the Master Onto Core only with the consensus certified new representations
(e) Validation of the Enhanced Master Onto Core

In the rest of this chapter we explain an approach for achieving the above requirements for Ontology Evolution.

6.2 "Living/Live" Onto-core to Support On-line Evolution

The original Nong's D/P system for mobile-clinic applications is static in the sense that the TCM onto-core does not evolve to keep abreast of advances in scientific findings. The first step to transform the static skeletal ontology into the "living/live" form is *automatic semantic aliasing* (ASA) [JWong08d]. The data structure to support the transformation and thus real-time ontology evolution is the Master Aliases Table (MAT), which is separated into two parts (Fig. 6.1):

(a) Part A: This is a direct transformation of the static skeletal ontological knowledge from the static side.
(b) Part B: This is for storing newly mined information by the text miner(s) from the open sources that include the open web and other conventional repertoires.

Conceptually, it is correct to say that in the next/new round of manual consensus certification the following holds: $PartA = PartA + PartB$. Every consensus certification round would involve sufficient number of domain experts, who would prune and decide what new knowledge items data-mined from the open sources should be included in the updated skeletal ontology.

The operation of a D/P system supported by a living TCM onto-core normally has the following basic steps:

(a) Initialization: This when the ASA transformation takes place.
(b) Data mining: Text mining is a form of data mining that suits the TCM domain, which is largely textual. The text miner ploughs the open sources and deposits the newly found knowledge into Part B of the MAT. The text miner(s) can be disconnected from Part B, which can be disconnected from Part A. The D/P system with part B disconnected falls back to the traditional static functionality.
(c) Automatic semantic aliasing: The ASA mechanism is non-stop and associates the newly data-mined knowledge in Part B with the original skeletal knowledge.

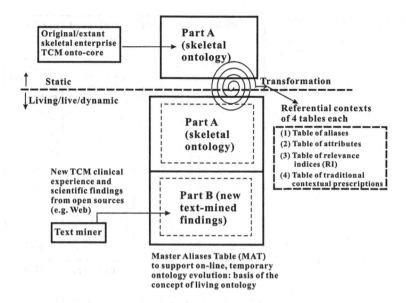

Fig. 6.1 Data structures to support the living ontology concept

In core of the ASA, mechanism is to compute the degree of similarity between two entities. For example, $A(x_1, x_2)$ and $B(x_1, x_3)$ mean that the entities A and B are defined by two separate sets of attributes, (x_1, x_2) and (x_1, x_3) respectively. These two entities are semantically similar because they have the common parameter x_1. In the ASA context, two entities are semantically the same if there are defined by exactly the same set of parameters, and they became aliases to each other if they were redefined later by only some common attributes such as x_1. In this sense the two entities $A(x_1, x_2)$ and $B(x_1, x_3)$ are associated by common parameter x_1. In the TCM domain, this kind of aliases is rife because the same illness, which was canonically enshrined in ancient formal classics, may be redefined by some different parameters due to geographical and epidemiological needs and differences. For example, if A was canonically enshrined (i.e. a canonical term or context) and now regarded as the reference (or referential context), then B is its alias. If both A and B are canonical, the context not being taken as the referential one is the alias. The ASA mechanism computes the degree of similarity or relevance index (RI) of an alias to the reference context (e.g. the similarity or RI of A to B if the latter is regarded as referential context). The computation of RI value depends on the algorithm adopted at the time. Since the local TCM onto-core of a Nong's D/P system variant was customized from the master enterprise onto-core, which is canonical in nature (constructed by consensus certification from formal TCM text, treatises, and case histories), all its entities are canonical. But, this local TCM

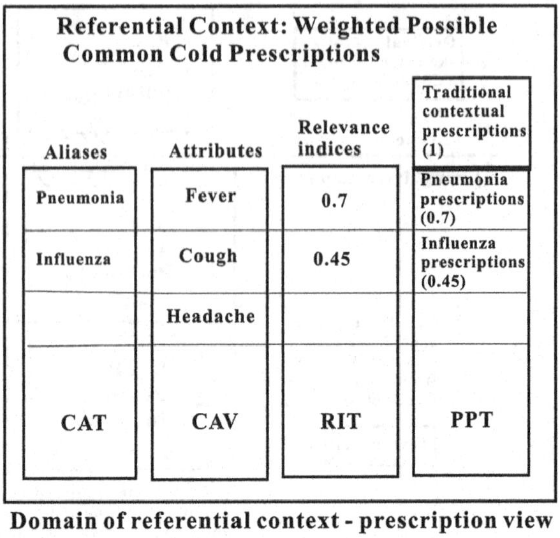

Fig. 6.2 A referential context
of four tables

Referential Context: Weighted Possible Common Cold Prescriptions			
Aliases	Attributes	Relevance indices	Traditional contextual prescriptions (1)
Pneumonia	Fever	0.7	Pneumonia prescriptions (0.7)
Influenza	Cough	0.45	Influenza prescriptions (0.45)
	Headache		
CAT	CAV	RIT	PPT

Domain of referential context - prescription view

onto-core risks the danger of stagnation with ancient canonical TCM knowledge, for it is not equipped to evolve automatically with time. The proposed ASA mechanism removes this danger by absorbing contemporary TCM information that includes new treatment cases by physicians and scientific reports uploaded to the open web. This kind of new knowledge can only be found with the help of text mining (TM), in an incessant, real-time manner.

We can generalize the evolution cycle in light of the consensus certification process by $A_i = A_{i-1} + B(pruned)$; where i denotes the current contents of the skeletal ontology A, and the Part B includes all the newly but "un-pruned" portion of the text-mined knowledge before A_i. More precisely A_i is "Part A of today after the manual evolution or consensus certification" and A_{i-1} is "Part A of yesterday". It is important to note that in light of the A_{i-1} skeletal ontology, Part B is initially empty at time equal to zero or t_0.

Every referential context or illness identified from the master enterprise ontology is supported by a data structure of four tables (Fig. 6.2): context aliases table (CAT) for aliases, context attributes table (CAV) for attributes, relevance indices table (RIT) for the relevance indices, and possible prescription table (PPT) for the traditional contextual prescriptions. All the attributes are weighted by domain experts during the consensus certification process to facilitate the computation of the RIs.

6.3 Knowledge and Experience Absorption

Knowledge and experience absorption or re-absorption in the TCM infrastructure described in this chapter includes standard printed text, non-standard printed text, and handwritten text. The sources of the knowledge to be re-absorbed into Part B of the Master Aliases Table (MAT) data structure that supports "living ontology" concept are ubiquitous in nature. They include old TCM classics, folklore, case histories of various geographical origins, and new scientific findings. For example, the Nong's D/P system accumulates the repertoire of patients' cases under the name of the same registered TCM physician, since his/her medical service under the Nong's mobile-clinic (MC) umbrella. With respect to Fig. 6.3 the registered (with the Hong Kong SAR Medical Council) physician "Allan" (00767) was assigned to one of the Nong's mobile clinic [Chinese Medicine Vehicle (CMV)] one day. Immediately all Allan's clinical experience including all the past patients' cases would be retrieved from the Nong's central database and loaded into a special area called "Experience Window". If Allan has worked for Nong's for the past twenty years, then all the relevant experience of Allan's since day one would be included. If there has been j number of identifiable physicians (X) in Nong's, then the accumulated clinical knowledge/experience from the j physicians is $CK_n = \sum_{j=1}^{n} X_j$. In fact, the text-miner would data-mine the CK_n contents in the same manner as for the open web. The text-mined knowledge is first stored in an intermediate format called the "index table". Then the ASA mechanism would transform them into "Part B", which is attached as an appendage to the "Part A" equivalent portion in the MAT contents. Physically the MAT has two parts (Fig. 6.3): the minimum Part A, which is logically the same as the "original/ untransformed" Part A, and the disposable Part B. Some of the Part B contents would become the new Part A contents after the next round of consensus

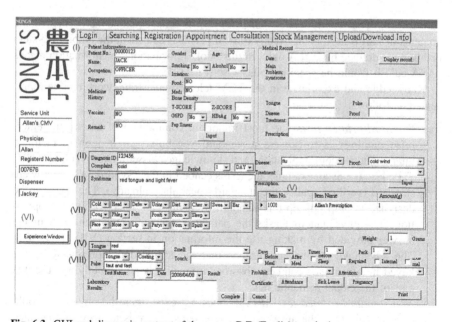

Fig. 6.3 GUI and diagnosis capture of the extant D/P (English version)

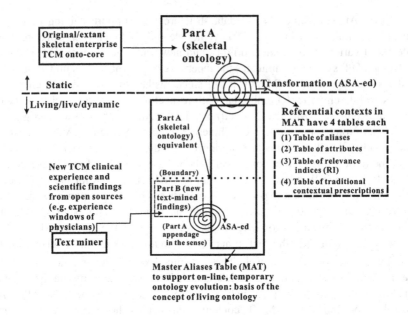

Fig. 6.4 Real-time information transformation ("ASA-ed") for MAT storage

certification. That is, $A_i = A_{i-1} + B(pruned)$; at time equal to zero (i.e. t_0) the contents of Part B in A_i is nil. At any time, if part B is detached, the ambit of system operation is defined by Part A only. In this book, information transformation means "ASA-ed"; it would be specified otherwise (Fig. 6.4).

Knowledge and experience in the TCM telemedicine framework can be represented as follows:

(a) *Standard printed text:* The most important connotation of having the enterprise ontology is to possess a standard vocabulary or lexicon to facilitate unambiguous communication and knowledge dissemination [Gruber93a]. Take Fig. 6.3 as an example, the terms echoed in the "Syndrome" window are standard (verified against the standard vocabulary already). The GUI can be designed to help upkeep this standard by using the "selective key-in" operation. The physician first asks the patient a question, and then keys in the answer provided by making use the information in section (VII) of Fig. 6.3. The advantage of this approach is that the knowledge represented by the keyed-in information can be reabsorbed immediately and directly because it is part of the extant semantic net.

(b) *Non-standard printed text:* If (VII) does not exist, then the physician would have to pen-input the answers by the patients. There is no way to guarantee that these pen-input are standard because it may include regional slangs. As a result, the keyed-in knowledge cannot be absorbed immediately and directly by the system because it may not be part of the extant semantic net and thus the ontology.

(c) *Handwritten text:* The imprecision of handwritten text is higher than the non-standard printed text. However, TCM has existed for many thousand years before the advent of computers, and old patients' cases are all hand-written based. As a result, re-absorption of old experience in the handwritten form requires special techniques.

6.4 Enablement of Easy Knowledge Reabsorption and Evolution

Knowledge reabsorption by any ontology is achieved through the consensus certification process. This process can be summarized by $O_i = O_{i-1} + NW$, where O_i is the ontology produced by the ith consensus certification cycle and NW is the pruned new knowledge accumulated since the $(i-1)$th cycle. The consensus certification process is usual manual and involves a sufficient number of domain experts. As a result, the pruned NW has to be incorporated into the ontology of the desired level, which can be:

(a) Global: It deals with syllogism (validity) and facts in a mixed manner.
(b) Enterprise: It is a subset of the global ontology isolated for enterprise-wide operation. It usually deals with facts, for example, the ontology defines the ambit of operation for an enterprise-based telemedicine system.
(c) Local: It is a subset or variant of an enterprise system, customized to suit the specific environments of operations.

Since the ontological information can be annotated by an appropriate metadata system, information can be added or deleted in the process of consensus certification. The annotating metadata system is separate from the essential/core ontological information, which can be expressed in any natural language (e.g. Chinese, English, Russia, etc.) or a mixture of them. For example, Fig. 6.5 is an excerpt of the Nong's enterprise TCM ontology in Chinese. This ontology is annotated by the three W3C languages in an "inter-nest-able" manner.

6.4.1 "Living Ontology" Aids Knowledge Absorption and Evolution

There are three main features in the concept of "live/living ontology" as follows: (i) automatic semantic aliasing (ASA); (ii) master aliases table (MAT); and (iii) matching IT (information technology) formalism with domain formalism is a commutable manner.

```
<?xml version="1.0" encoding="big5" ?        /* Chinese only */>
<!DOCTYPE              rdf:RDF               [<!ENTITY              xsd
"http://www.w3.org/2001/XMLSchema#">]>
  <rdf:RDF
        xmlns:rdf="http://www.w3.org/1999/02/22-rdf-syntax-ns#"
        xmlns:rdfs="http://www.w3.org/2000/01/rdf-schema#"
        xmlns:xsd="http://www.w3.org/2001/XMLSchema#"
        xmlns:tcm="c:/testSchema#"
        xml:base="file:///./#">
        <tcm:病名 rdf:ID="感冒" />
        <tcm:證型 rdf:ID="風寒證">
              <rdfs:subClassOf rdf:resource="#感冒"/>
              <tcm:兼證 rdf:ID="風寒證兼證">口不渴或渴喜熱飲</tcm:兼
證>

              <tcm:舌苔 rdf:ID="風寒證舌苔">舌苔薄白</tcm:舌苔>
              <tcm:脈象 rdf:ID="風寒證脈象">脈象浮或兼緊</tcm:脈象>
        </tcm:證型>
        <tcm:主證 rdf:ID="風寒證主證">
              <rdfs:subClassOf rdf:resource="#風寒證"/>
        </tcm:主證>
        <tcm:衛表 rdf:ID="風寒證衛表">
              <rdfs:subClassOf rdf:resource="#風寒證主證"/>
              <tcm:怕冷 rdf:ID="風寒證怕冷">怕冷重</tcm:怕冷>
              <tcm:發熱 rdf:ID="風寒證發熱">發熱輕</tcm:發熱>
```

Fig. 6.5 An excerpt of a TCM onto-core

The ASA concept associates two entities by their degree of similarity or relevance. It is the IT expression/formalism: $P(Ter_1 \cup Ter_2) = P(Ter_1) + P(Ter_2) - P(Ter_1 \cap Ter_2)$. The symbols $\cup$ and $\cap$ stand for union and intersection respectively. $P(Ter_1 \cap Ter_2)$, which is the probability for $(Ter_1 \cap Ter_2)$, is the relevance index (RI) that measures the similarity between the two terms Ter_1 and Ter_2. If these two terms are 100 % similar (the same), then they are logically-equivalent synonyms. If the $Ter_1 \neq Ter_2$ (i.e. not logically equivalent) is true; then Ter_1 and Ter_2 are aliases only (not synonyms). $P(Ter_1)$ and $P(Ter_2)$ are the probabilities for the multi-representations (other meanings).

To apply the IT formalism $P(Ter_1 \cup Ter_2)$ in the TCM domain, it must match a particular formalism or principle in the domain seamlessly and in a commutable manner. By commutable, it means that the experts in two different domains (e.g. IT and TCM) see the same conceptual essence unambiguously. For example, if we match the IT formalism with the universal TCM SIMILARITY/SAME (i.e. "同") formalism (i.e. "同病異治, 異病同治" in classical TCM terminology [WHO07]). The outcome of combining IT and TCM formalism in a commutable meaner is the association of relevant knowledge, which may have appeared disjoint on the surface. For example, the IT formalism associates four patient cases in Fig. 6.6, and these cases may came from different physicians of different geographical regions. In the regions a, b, and c, the name of the illness is the same, namely A. For region x, the name of the illness (i.e. X) differs. Yet, these four cases have the common symptoms x_1 and x_3. From the concept of referential context (RC) in the living ontology framework [JWong09d], with respect to the Illness (A, a) as the RC, the different cases Illness (A, b), Illness (A, c), and Illness (X, x) have different relevance indices (RI). The computation of RI values for any setup (e.g. enterprise setup) is the result of the current consensus certification process.

We can put Fig. 6.6 into perspective by assuming, for example, that the three cases Illness (A, a), Illness (A, b) and Illness (A, c) have different prescriptions, namely PAa, PAb and PAc respectively. From the SIMILARITY/SAME principle the total/common set of usable prescriptions for treating the three cases should be conceptually $P_{all} = PAa \cup PAb \cup PAc$. The $\cup$ operation (i.e. union) associates the three different prescriptions into a single pool (i.e. the common set P_{all}) by identifying the common attributes or factors. In fact, it is normal for the same illness to be defined by some different attributes on top of the common set, due to the geographical and epidemiological disparities. Yet, the meaning of efficacy of P_{all} with respect to every RC differs because the RI values for namely PAa, PAb and PAc with respect to every RC are not the same.

The $P_{all} = PAa \cup PAb \cup PAc$ concept is an important basis to aid knowledge absorption and evolution. The ontology of an operation system is living if this concept is realized in a real-time manner—a living ontology. Certainly, some cases based on $P_{all} = PAa \cup PAb \cup PAc$ may be pruned in the new round of manual consensus certification. This is inevitable if an enterprise wants to define its ambit of operation clearly.

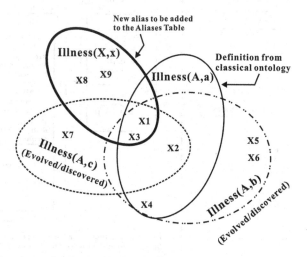

Fig. 6.6 Illness (X, x) is an alias to the Illness (A, a) RC

6.5 Coherent Consensus-Certified Knowledge Engineering

In the living ontology framework, coherent consensus-certified knowledge engineering is semi-automatic. The knowledge engineering process can be better
explained by using the master aliases table (MAT) in Fig. 6.7.

The living ontology is supported by the information management activities in the
MAT as shown in Fig. 6.7. The enterprise ontology is abstracted by two forms here:

(a) Enterprise vocabulary or {V}: This contains all the names of entity in the
enterprise ontology but not their associations within the ontological subsumption hierarchy.
(b) Semantic net: This is the middle layer of any ontology-based system (e.g.
UMLS [UMLS]) in the context of this book for machine understanding and
processing (i.e. parsing).

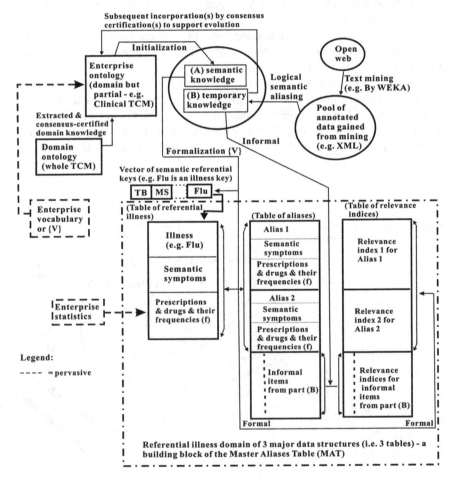

Fig. 6.7 Three main data vectors/tables per RC illness in the MAT

According to the meta-interface concept, any ontology-based system can be automatically generated from the given iconic specification. This specification is a collection of icons and each icon is a semantic path embedded in the ontological subsumption hierarchy in the given master ontology (Fig. 6.8). If the given master ontology is updated, the same iconic specification will generated the updated target system.

Referring to Fig. 6.7 the semantic knowledge in part (A) is static in the sense that it is the last consensus-certified version. Part (B) represents the newly acquired knowledge from open sources and this knowledge is not consensus-certified at all, as shown in Fig. 6.1. Advancing the old part (A) to a new part (A) by the process of consensus certification can be represented logically by $onto_{i+1} = onto_i + P\_part(B)$, where: (i) $onto_{i+1}$ is the new part (A); (ii) $onto_i$ is the old part (A); and (iii) $P\_part(B)$ is the pruned information from the temporary part (B). There is nil contents in the temporary part (B) when $onto_{i+1}$ has just come into existence. Therefore, the MAT facilitates coherent consensus-certified knowledge engineering by accumulating relevant useful information into the temporary part (B) in a real-time manner.

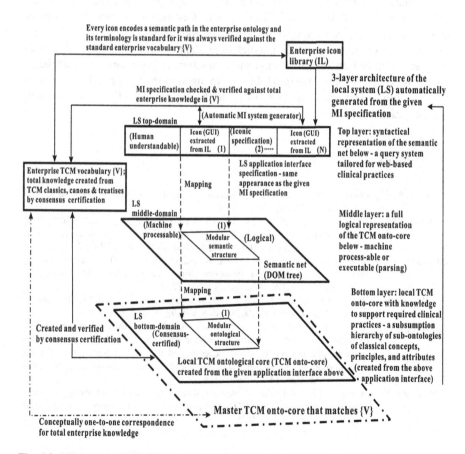

Fig. 6.8 MI concept—EOD-ISD mechanism

The relationship between part (A) and part (B) lies in the concept of referential context (RC), and in this case an RC is always the illness identified from part (A). Every RC (e.g. flu) in the MAT has three relevant tables: (i) illness table that contains relevant information such as semantic symptoms, standard prescriptions and their use frequencies; (ii) table of aliases that has two parts: consensus-certified aliases transformed directly from part (A) by the ASA (automatic semantic aliasing) mechanism; and new aliases (not consensus-certified) data-mined from open sources in a real-time fashion; and (iii) table of relevance indices (RI) that indicate the degrees of similarity (i.e. $P(Ter_1 \cap Ter_2)$) between the aliases and the RC (e.g. flu in Fig. 6.7). The MAT implementation is an open issue; it can be centralized or distributed/pervasive depending on the operation environment.

6.6 Recapitulation

In this chapter, we addressed the issue of TCM Ontology Evolution. The need for TCM Ontology evolution arises from several factors including scientific advances, new disease types, new clinical prescriptions and treatment regimes. There are several aspects to ontology evolution including identification of new knowledge, its representation, consensus certification and evaluation. A systematic approach based on the use of the Master Aliasing Table is explained in this chapter. This approach has been implemented and is used to update the Master Onto Core that is widely used in practice.

References

[Gruber93a]   Gruber, T.R.: A translation approach to portable ontology specification. Knowl. Acquisition 5(2), 199–220 (1993)
[Khattak09]   Khattak, A.M., Latif, K, Lee, S.Y. and Lee, Y.K.: Ontology evolution: a survey and future challenges. In: The 2nd International Conference on u- and e-Service, Science and Technology (UNESST09), Jeju, Korea, 10–12 Dec 2009
[Stojanovic02]   Stojanovic, L., Madche, A., Motik, B. and Stojanovic, N.: User driven ontology evolution management. In: European Conference on Knowledge Engineering and Management (EKAW), pp. 285–300, (2002)
[WHO07]   WHO: International Standard Terminologies on Traditional Medicine in the Western Pacific Region (2007). ISBN 978-92-9061-248-7
[JWong08d]   Wong, J.H.K., Lin, W.W.K. and Wong, A.K.Y.: Real-time enterprise ontology evolution to aid effective clinical telemedicine with text mining and automatic semantic aliasing support. In: Proceedings of the 7th International Conference on Ontologies, Databases, and Applications of Semantics (ODBASE), Monterey, Mexico, 11–13 Nov 2008
[JWong09d]   Wong, J.H.K.: PhD thesis: web-based data mining and discovery of useful herbal ingredients (**WD²UHI**), Department of Computing, Hong Kong Polytechnic University (2009)

Chapter 7
TCM Telemedicine Infrastructure

7.1 Introduction

The Nong's mobile clinics (MC) provide a successful example of telemedicine in the TCM domain. As a Telemedicine System, it needs an appropriate and effective infrastructure to deliver the required services remotely. Figure 7.1 shows a typical system architecture for such a Telemedicine system.

The "diagnosis/prescription (D/P)" system that supports the MC has been treating hundreds of patients in the Hong Kong SAR since its deployment 4 years ago.

The mobile Internet supports both wireless and wireline communications. One of the comprehensive ways to depict this support is the "surrogate" model [JWong09d] shown in Fig. 7.2.

Many clients are served by many dedicated proxy servers called the surrogates. These clients may be grouped so that they can be matched with the dedicated surrogate server. This surrogate model is basically a "terminal system model (TSM)."

The Nong's D/P telemedicine system is an example of how the TSM works. The client in the Nong's case is the mobile clinic, and the small form device (SFF) is the notebook on board the vehicle. The physician usually treats the patients locally and communicates with the surrogate. The dedicated surrogate that serves the physician, who is a member of a pre-assigned group, tries to serve the request quickly and correctly. It asks for peer surrogates within Nong's and sometimes other known collaborators outside to help under certain conditions as explained in Sect. 7.3.

7.2 Performance Modelling of the Pervasive TCM Telemedicine Infrastructure on the Mobile Internet

As mentioned earlier the mobile Internet supports both wireless and wireline communications. We use the "surrogate" model [JWong09d] to depict this support as shown in Fig. 7.2. Many clients (e.g. Traditional Chinese Medicine (TCM)

© Springer-Verlag Berlin Heidelberg 2015
A.K.Y. Wong et al., *Semantically Based Clinical TCM Telemedicine Systems*,
Studies in Computational Intelligence 587, DOI 10.1007/978-3-662-46024-5_7

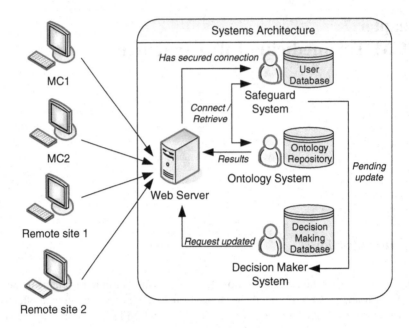

Fig. 7.1 Schematic representation of TCM telemedicine infrastructure

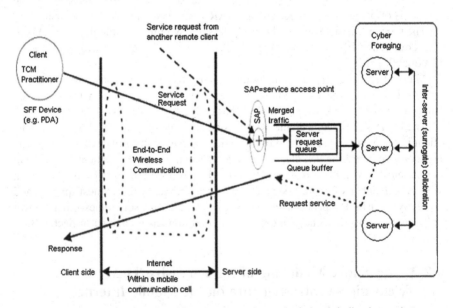

Fig. 7.2 Client-server surrogate model supporting end-to-end wireless/wireline interactions

practitioners) are served by many dedicated proxy servers called the surrogates. These clients may be grouped so that they can be matched with the dedicated surrogate server. From an analytic point of view, the surrogate model is basically a "terminal system model (TSM)" or "machine interference model" [Mitrani87] that can be depicted by Figs. 7.3 and 7.4, and its corresponding Markov chain that depicts the system dynamics in Fig. 7.5. In Fig. 7.4, λ and μ are respectively the mean service request input rate and service rate. Therefore, $1/\lambda$ is the average think time; $1/\mu$ the execution time; and $\rho = (\lambda/\mu) \leq 1$ the system utilization. Figure 7.5 generalizes three cases of system of system dynamic (although it is present for case 2) as follows:

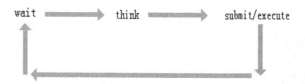

Fig. 7.3 A simplified/generalized TSM

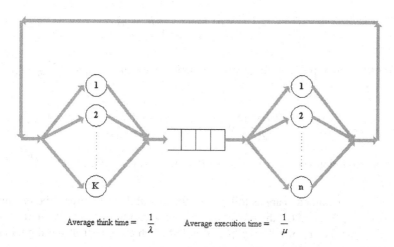

Fig. 7.4 The more detailed TSM model

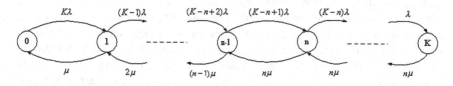

Fig. 7.5 General Markov chain for Fig. 7.4

Case 1: $(K - j + 1)\lambda P_{j-1} = j\mu P_j$;   for $j = 1, 2, 3, \ldots, K$

Case 2: $(K - j + 1)\lambda P_{j-1} = j\mu P_j$;   for $j = 1, 2, 3, \ldots, n - 1$

Case 3: $(K - j + 1)\lambda P_{j-1} = n\mu P_j$;   for $j = n, n + 1, \ldots, n - 1$

For the $K \leq n$ condition, case 1 applies and the state equation for the queue dynamics becomes

$$P_j = \frac{K!}{(K - j)!j!} \rho^j P_0.$$

From the probability function $\sum_{j=0}^{K} P_j = \sum \rho^j P_0 = 1$ the following holds:

(i) $P_0 = \left[\sum_{j=0}^{j=k} \frac{K!\rho^j}{(K-j)!j!} \right]^{-1}$

(ii) $P_j = \dfrac{\frac{K!\rho^j}{(K-j)!j!}}{\sum_{j=0}^{K} \left[\frac{K!\rho^j}{(K-j)!j!} \right]}$

In fact, P_j can be transformed into the equation below:

$$P_j = \binom{K}{j}\rho^j \Big/ \sum_{j=0}^{K} \left[\binom{K}{j}\rho^j \right]$$

From the view point of the following series, we can conclude $\sum_{j=0}^{K} [\binom{K}{j}\rho^j] = (1 + \rho)^K$:

$$(1 + \rho)^K = 1 + K\rho + \frac{K(K - 1)}{2!}\rho^2 + \cdots + \frac{K(K - 1).\ldots.(K - n - 1)}{n!}K^n + \cdots$$

Thus, equation be rewritten as: $P_j = \binom{K}{j}\rho^j \big/ (1 + \rho)^K$ or $P_j = \binom{K}{j}(\frac{\rho^j}{(1+\rho)^j})$ $(\frac{1}{(1+\rho)})^{K-1}$

The useful parameters are as follows: (i) the probability of a user to be in a think state is $1/(1 + \rho)$; and (ii) the probability of a server to be busy is $\rho/(1 + \rho)$. From these two parameters, the throughput of a TSM, which is basically a digital eco-system [Hadzic07], can be represented as $T = \mu K \rho/(1 - \rho)$.

The different TSM models (Figs. 7.2, 7.3, 7.4 and 7.5) do not really take the Internet channel latency into account. For example, in end-to-end wireless communication, there could be many retransmissions due to the channel error σ_w. Meanwhile, the surrogate, which should take care of the particular user group, may collaborate with other peer surrogates for various reasons. Then, in light of the client/surrogate (C/S) path, the channel error probability is σ_S, which includes σ_w. The possible C/S service roundtrip latency can be defined in terms of σ_S and the *average number of trails* (ANT) to get a transmission success as $ANT = \sum_{j=1}^{N} j P_j$;

P_j is the chance for success at the jth trial, defined as $P_j = \sigma_S^{j-1}(1 - \sigma_s)$. Therefore, $ANT = \sum_{j=1}^{N} jP_j$ can be redefined as $ANT = \sum_{j=1}^{N \to \infty} j[\sigma_S^{j-1}(1 - \sigma_S)] \approx 1/(1 - \sigma_S)$. Any dynamic problems along the C/S path, for example, sudden on-line changes in Internet traffic pattern [JWong08e], would increase σ_S and lengthen the service roundtrip time (RTT). Figure 7.2 is a typical pervasive architecture for building any digital ecosystems such as the Nong's diagnosis/prescription (D/P) system for mobile-clinic application. This vehicle-based D/P system, since its successful deployment 4 years ago, has been treating hundreds of patients in the Hong Kong SAR alone.

7.3 Realization Example

The Nong's D/P telemedicine system is an example of how the TSM represented by Fig. 7.2 is realized. The client in the Nong's case is the mobile clinic, and the SFF (small form device is the notebook on board the vehicle. The physician usually treats the patients locally and communicates with the surrogate under the following conditions: (i) drug replenishment request; (ii) report of signs of a possible epidemic outbreak; (iii) solicitation of second opinions for unusual cases; and (iv) drug toxicity control. The dedicated surrogate that serves the physician, who is a member of a pre-assigned group, tires its own best to serve the request quickly and correctly. It asks for peer surrogates within Nong's and sometimes other known collaborators outside for help under the following conditions:

(a) The surrogate is too busy: It changes its original M/M/1 status to the M/M/n parallel operation. As a result a service speedup (S) is attained, defined as $S = W_1/W_n = (1 - \rho/n)/(1 - \rho)$; where W_1 is the response time for M/M/1; W_2 is the response time for M/M/n; and ρ is the system utilization. The surrogate can be very busy because it serves many clients, which may be connected by both wireless and wireline means. All the service requests merge at the surrogate service access point (SAP) in an exponential manner. If the requests are not served fast enough, then the possible surrogate buffer overflow may increase σ_S and thus ANT.

(b) The surrogate lacks the required knowledge: It has to solicit help from others.

The series screen captures, namely, Figs. 7.6, 7.7, 7.8 and 7.9 represent a real D/P system operation, which was based on a "thin" personal digital assistant (PDA). This customized version of the Nong's TCM D/P system is called the TCM Pervasive Digital HealthCare System (T-PDHS). The PDA is "thin", for it has limited memory and has to load its patient records from the central database management via its dedicated surrogate proxy. In Fig. 7.6, the physician activated the PDA with its account number and password. Figure 7.7 shows the screen for patient record retrieval. If the physician activated the "Prescription" icon/button, then the prescription screen would be displayed (Fig. 7.8). Part of the "PDA/surrogate" Internet

Fig. 7.6 T-PDHS login
screen

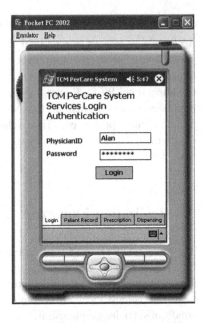

Fig. 7.7 T-PDHS patient
record

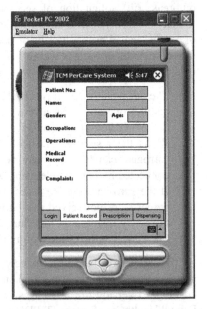

channel traffic was shown by Fig. 7.9, and the off-line analysis of this traffic trace or
time series by the Selfis tool [Karagiannis02] indicates that it is LRD in nature. LRD
includes both heavy-tailed and self-similar bursts; the latter could cause serious
service roundtrip time delay or even temporary channel blackout [Lin07].

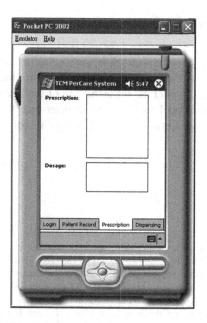

Fig. 7.8 T-PDHS prescription screen

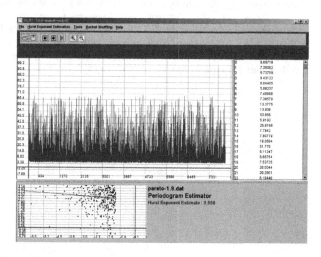

Fig. 7.9 LRD—Periodogram estimator in *Selfis*

7.4 Recapitulation

The TCM Telemedicine System requires an appropriate infrastructure to enable the delivery of the required services. In this chapter, we utilize the surrogate model and terminal system model to model the infrastructure of the Telemedicine system. We next present a Markov Model that is used to determine the performance of the infrastructure. Lastly, we show a practical realization of this and the captured performance.

References

[Hadzic07]   Hadzic, M., Chang, E., Dillon, T.S.: Methodology framework for the design of digital ecosystems. In: SMC, pp. 7–12 (2007)

[Karagiannis02] Karagiannis, T., Faloutsos, M.: SELFIS: a tool for self-similarity and long-range dependence analysis. In: 1st Workshop on fractals and self-similarity in data mining: issues and approaches (IN KDD), July 2002

[Lin07]   Lin, W.W.K., Wong, A.K.Y., Dillon, T.S., Chang, E.: Detection of Fractal Breakdowns by the Novel Real-Time Pattern Detection Model (Enhanced-RTPD+ Holder Exponent) for Web Applications. ISORC, pp. 79–86 (2007)

[Mitrani87]   Mitrani, I.: Modelling of Computer and Communication Systems, CUP, p. 114 (1987). ISBN 0521314224

[JWong08e]   Wong, J.H.K., Lin, W.W.K., Wong, A.K.Y., Dillon, T.S.: Applying neuro-fuzzy dynamic buffer tuning to make web-based telemedicine successful. In: Proceedings of the International Conference on E-business and Telecommunication Networks (ICETE), Porto, Portugal, 26–29 July 2008

[JWong09d]   Wong, J.H.K.: Web-based data mining and discovery of useful herbal ingredients (WD2UHI). PhD. thesis, Department of Computing, Hong Kong Polytechnic University (2009)

Chapter 8
Recapitulation and Future Directions

8.1 Introduction

In this chapter, we provide a summary of the main findings of the Work on the Intelligent TCM Telemedicine System described in this book. After that, we proceed to discuss future directions for the research and development of the TCM System.

8.2 Recapitulation

In the first chapter, we explored the issues which created the need for an Intelligent Traditional Chinese Medicine (TCM) Telemedicine System. Specifically we identified the following characteristics of such a system namely:

1. Knowledge consultation
2. Curative aspects
3. Training by e-learning
4. Management and control
5. Efficient and reliable information communication technology (ICT) support
6. Explicit semantics

As this book is focused on the scientific and engineering issues that underpin the building of a semantically-based clinical TCM telemedicine system, it must explore the usefulness of ontology in the building of computer-aided TCM systems; choice of the tool for modeling the ontology blueprint layout; TCM telemedicine infrastructure and mobile clinics and how telemedicine system building can be automated with quality assurance, and how a telemedicine system can be deployed over the web.

This required that we addressed the following issues in the work namely:

(a) Ontology modelling
(b) Ontology implementation tool

© Springer-Verlag Berlin Heidelberg 2015
A.K.Y. Wong et al., *Semantically Based Clinical TCM Telemedicine Systems*,
Studies in Computational Intelligence 587, DOI 10.1007/978-3-662-46024-5_8

(c) Internet capability
d) Architecture and cross-layer logical transitivity
(e) Automatic system generation
(f) Pervasive support
(g) Ontology evolution

These were each addressed in turn in the subsequent chapters of the book.

A key aspect of the system design is the three layer Architectural framework. This consists of a:

- Bottom Layer—The bottom layer is the knowledge/database that embeds the subsumption hierarchy that represents the logical relationships among the physical data items/entities included in the consensus-certified ontology.
- Middle Layer—This subsumption hierarchy is also realized in the middle layer as the semantic net for machine understanding and execution.
- Top Layer—The top layer is the query system that implements the ontology for user understanding and manipulation.

These three have cross-layer semantic transitivity. With this transitivity any entity in any layer should have corresponding representations in the other two layers.

In order to properly ensure this cross layer transitivity across various distributed realizations of the system, we utilize automatic system generation or customization (ASG/C). This approach is, in fact, a new software engineering paradigm, which requires the user to provide the ontology blueprint layout. With support of the master ontology, where the ontology specification is either a part or the whole of it, the ASG/C mechanism generates/customizes the final ontology-based system.

The Intelligent TCM telemedicine system needs the support of a wireless-based pervasive computing infrastructure, which maintains the smart spaces for the collaborating systems. In the PuraPharm mobile-clinics environment, the collaborating systems are the mobile clinics. The Pervasive Computing Infrastructure maintains the smart space occupied by a mobile clinic (MC) which communicates with the central system, as well as its peers, via the wireless means. The MC operation is semi-autonomous because the physician can treat the patient at the spot, but the case history of the patient may have to be downloaded from the central computer that runs the fast network.

To ensure the TCM Ontology does not become frozen and outdated, it must be able to absorb information and knowledge from every fresh case into the "master" ontology as new knowledge. Hence, it is clear that there is a need for a framework of Ontology evolution for the TCM ontology so that it reflects the new knowledge and insights.

To achieve ontology evolution we need to:

- Ascertain the new knowledge—This is done by text mining.
- Represent this potential new knowledge temporarily in a form compatible with Ontology—A temporary representation of these potential new knowledge is stored in a part of the Master Aliasing Table.

- Carryout Consensus Certification of this new potential new knowledge.
- Enhancing the Master Ontology only with the Consensus Certified portions of the new knowledge.

8.3 Future Work

There are 5 directions in which the Intelligent TCM Telemedicine system can be enhanced and extended. These directions are as follows, namely:

1. Use of Collaborative Multi Agents to support the interpretation of Chinese Medicine Queries and Diagnosis
2. Integrative Medicine
3. Cyber Physical Systems or The Internet of things.
4. Cloud Computing
5. Conjoint Structured and Unstructured Data Mining

These are discussed in turn below.

8.3.1 Collaborative Multi Agent Recommender Systems

The TCM Ontology developed in this research helps address the need for communication among different TCM Practitioners using a common and sharable set of concepts and relationships and a common vocabulary. In its use in practice in the field by mobile clinics and medical clinics, it has been found to be effective in clarifying misunderstandings regarding concepts, relationships and project information. The TCM Ontology defines common shareable TCM knowledge representing concepts: what the concepts are, how they are related, and why they are related. Due to the nature of the Ontology as a passive structure, as are many Ontologies that exist on the Web including the TCM Ontology, it is most effective in providing support if the end-users know exactly what concepts and relationships they are referring to. However, sometimes the users are unable to identify or articulate the precise concepts they wish to access in a form consonant with the TCM Ontology. In these situations, it would be useful to have active support which take a vaguely formulated query related to a problem the end user needs to address. The development of a recommender approach to provide active support and recommendations to TCM Practitioners that can effectively transform their vaguely formulated query into a precise ontology search would greatly enhance the usability of the system.

This will provide active support to a TCM Practitioner who comes with knowledge of an issue, rather than knowing precisely which concepts and relationships he/she needs clarification on. A good way to provide this support is through the use of collaborative recommender multi agents who capture and represent knowledge that allows mapping of issues onto the Ontology.

8.3.2 Integrative Medicine

Increasingly western allopathic medical practitioners are utilizing TCM Herbs or techniques in conjunction with the allopathic drugs. While this is a welcome development, it requires careful elaboration in its use. It is known that if more than one allopathic drug is used, drug interactions can produce one of the following situations:

1. The drugs have a positive and complementary effect on each other increasing their therapeutic capability.
2. They have a negative effect which reduces the potential effect of one or more of the drugs.
3. They can have an adverse reaction introducing further undesirable side effects.
4. They can have no effect on each other.

When using TCM Herbs with Orthodox allopathic drugs, one has to be aware that the above four interactions can also take place.

When we introduce the use of TCM Herbs with the orthodox allopathic, the situation can become more complex due to the fact that the TCM Medical model is somewhat different than the Allopathic model and hence it is necessary to get a more precise understanding of the pharmacology properties of TCM Herbs. In order to support this, we utilize a HerbMiners and give a HerbMiners Road Map in Fig. 8.1. Also increasingly the TCM area is seeing the development of TCM Herb granule based medications where the pharmacological medical properties are better controlled. See Fig. 8.2.

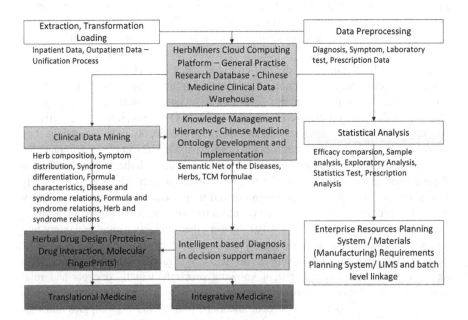

Fig. 8.1 HerbMiners R&D RoadMap

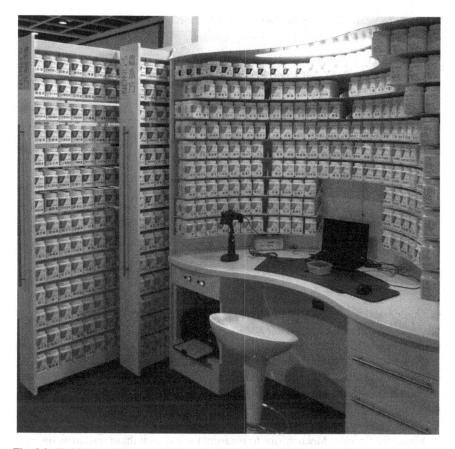

Fig. 8.2 HerbMiners Chinese medicine granule dispensing system

To help characterize the TCM herbs pharmacological and medicinal properties and relate them to an Allopathic equivalent actions, we suggest the use of a template such as that proposed in Table 8.1.

A Related development here is Structure Data Mining of herbs—升麻 Cimicifuga racemosa (Sheng Ma) by the HKU research team and our company (see Novel Compounds and Uses Thereof for Treating Inflammation and Modulating Immune Responses).

8.3.3 Cloud Computing for TCM Telemedicine

When one examines the key characteristics of Cloud Computing, one notices the following [Dillon10]:

Table 8.1 Integrative medicine template—to identify the effect and the interaction type

Paper code	DH-006
Pin Yin	Da Huang
Pharmaceutical name	Radix et Rhizoma Rhei
Common name	Rhubarb Root and Rhizome
Orthodox drug	Laxatives
Result/effect	Concurrent use may increase risk of hypokalemia
Reason	The herb is an anthraquinone-containing laxative itself. Long term abuse may lead to hepatitis, electrolyte disturbances (hypokalaemia, hypocalcaemia), metabolic acidosis, malabsorption, weight loss, albuminuria, and haematuria... etc.
Reference	World Health Organization. **WHO monographs on selected medicinal plants.** Vol. 1. Geneva: World Health Organization, 1999
Source	Herb-drug interaction handbook
Valid interaction?	Yes
Interaction type	Harmful

- On-demand self-service: Instantaneous need at a particular timeslot can avail computing resources in an automatic fashion.
- Broad network access: Computing resources are delivered over the network and used by various client applications.
- Resource pooling: Computing resources are "pooled" together to serve multiple consumers—multi-tenancy or virtualization
- Rapid elasticity: Resources become immediately available—can scale up whenever they want, and release them once finished to scale down.
- Measured Service: Mechanisms to measure the usage of these resources for each individual consumer through metering.

Cloud computing is a model for enabling convenient, on-demand network access to a shared pool of configurable computing resources (e.g., networks, servers, storage, applications, and services) that can be rapidly provisioned and released with minimal management effort or service provider interaction [Mell09]. Cloud Computing refers to both the applications delivered as services over the Internet and the hardware and systems software in the datacenters that provide those services [Armbrust09].

An important element of cloud computing is virtualization.

Several of the above features can be effectively utilized by the TCM Tele-medicine namely:

- Elasticity
    - No up-front commitment and contract—pay as you go
    - You use it whenever you want, and let it go once you finish
    - Scale up and down—computing on-demand
    - Scale horizontally—various services on-demand
    - Infinite, Immediate, and Invisible computing resources

- Service Level Agreement and QoS between individual clinics and the central computer
- Robust and reliable
- Ubiquitous access
- Unawareness of which resources being used
- Availability

8.3.4 Cyber Physical Systems and the Internet of Things for TCM Telemedicine

The recent development of Cyber-Physical Systems (CPS) provides a unified framework connecting the cyber world with the physical world. CPS allows for robust and flexible systems with multi-scale dynamics and integrated wired and wireless networking for managing the flows of mass, energy, and information in a coherent way through integration of computing and communication capabilities with the monitoring and/or control of entities in the physical world in a dependable, safe, secure, efficient and real-time fashion. CPS is a new research field seeking to integrate embedded real-time systems into the Internet. CPS is often long lasting, with 24×7 operations and must evolve without losing stability. CPS is a heterogeneous system of systems, consisting of computing devices, embedded systems, sensors and actuators that are inter-connected allowing for task execution linking the cyber world and the physical world.

An important application for CPS is future health care systems. These applications will require seamless and synergetic integration between sensing, computation, and control with physical devices and processes. Building CPS is not a trivial task. It requires a new ground-breaking theory that models cyber and physical resources in a unified framework. For example, many key requirements (e.g. uncertainty, inaccuracy, etc.) crucial to physical systems are not captured and fully dealt with in the computer science research agenda. In a similar vein, computational complexity, system evolution and software failure are often ignored from the physical theory viewpoint, which treats computation as a precise, error-free, static 'black-box'. The solution to CPS must transcend the boundary between the cyber world and the physical world by providing a unified infrastructure that permits integrated models addressing issues from both worlds simultaneously. One common thing with CPS is the real time monitoring, control and management of different activities. This:

- Is achieved by an appropriate Architectural Framework.
- Is achieved by an Event-based model [Singh12].
- Is achieved by a QoS-based model [Dillon11a].
- Is achieved by a Semantic-based model [Dillon12].
- Involves Big Data usually streaming at High rates.

Our focus, in this chapter, is on Telemedicine CPS systems that detect the occurrence of an emergency or deteriorating situation and take corrective actions to ameliorate or mitigate the consequences of these. For these systems, given their need for different computational capabilities in different contexts, we explore the use of an integrated CPS-Cloud Ecosystem to meet these needs effectively.

8.3.4.1 Brief Overview of Architectural Framework for CPS Systems

Our vision of CPS is as follows: networked information systems that are tightly coupled with the physical process and environment through a massive number of geographically distributed devices [Dillon11b]. As networked information systems, CPS involves computation, human activities, and automated decision making enabled by information and communication technology. More importantly, these computation, human activities and intelligent decisions are aimed at monitoring, controlling and integrating physical processes and environment to support operations and management in the physical world. The scale of such information systems ranges from micro-level, embedded systems to ultra-large systems of systems. Devices provide the basic interface between the cyber world and the physical one.

We have previously proposed a Web-of-Things (WoT) framework for CPS systems [Dillon11b] that argues the Internet-of-Things in order to deal with issues such as information-centric protocol, deterministic QoS, context-awareness, etc. We argue that substantial extra work such as our proposed WoT framework is required before IoT can be utilized to address technical challenges in CPS Systems that are capable of being used in TCM Telemedicine Systems.

The building block of WoT is REpresentational State Transfer (REST), which is a specific architectural style [NSF08]. It is, in effect, a refinement and constrained version of the architecture of the Web and the HTTP 1.1 protocol [Lee08], which has become the most successful large-scale distributed application that the world has known to date. Proponents of REST style argue that existing Remote Procedure Call (RPC)-based Web services architecture is indeed not "Web-oriented". Rather, it is merely the "Web" version of RPC, which is more suited to a closed local network, and has serious potential weakness when deployed across the Internet, particularly with regards to scalability, performance, flexibility, and implementability [Lee09].

The WoT framework for CPS is shown in Fig. 8.3, which consists of five layers— WoT Device, WoT Kernel, WoT Overlay, WoT Context and WoT API. Underneath the WoT framework is the cyber-physical interface (e.g. sensors, actuators, cameras) that interacts with the surrounding physical environment. The proposed WoT framework allows the cyber world to observe, analyse, understand, and control the physical world using these data to perform mission/time-critical tasks.

1. WoT Device: This layer constitute the cyber-physical interface of the system. It is a resource-oriented abstraction that unifies the management of various devices. It states the device semantics in terms of REST-ful protocol.

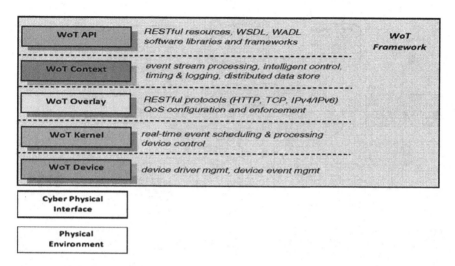

Fig. 8.3 WoT framework for CPS

2. WoT Kernel: This layer provides low level run-time for communication, scheduling, and WoT resources management. It identifies events and allocates the required resources, i.e. network bandwidth, processing power and storage capacity for dealing with a large amount of data from the WoT Device layer.
3. WoT Overlay: This layer is an application-driven, network-aware logical abstraction atop the current Internet infrastructure. It will manage volatile network behavior such as latency, data loss, jitter and bandwidth by allowing nodes to select paths with better and more predictable performance.
4. WoT Context: This layer provides semantics for events captured by the lower layers of WoT framework. This layer is also responsible for decision making and controlling the behavior of the CPS applications.
5. WoT API: This layer provides abstraction in the form of interfaces that allow developers to interact with the WoT framework.

Sensors, actuators, buildings, cities, vehicles, power grid, etc.

Based on the WoT framework in Fig. 8.3, the CPS reference architecture is shown in Fig. 8.4, which aims to capture both domain requirements and infrastructure requirements at a high level of abstraction. It is expected that CPS applications can be built atop the CPS reference architecture.

More details about the CPS Fabric structure and the CPS node structure are given in [Dillon11b].

8.3.4.2 Semantics for CPS Systems

A key aspect of CPS systems is representing the semantics of events and sensors. Event representation has to cater for the distributed real-time CPS. Events are one

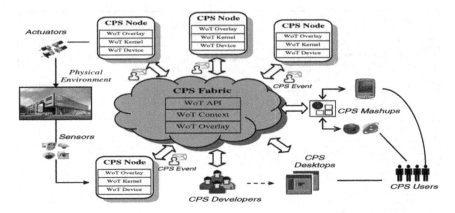

Fig. 8.4 CPS reference architecture

of the key initiators of activities in Cyber-Physical Systems. They provide a natural way to specify components of open systems in terms of interfaces and observable behaviour. Events can also form the basis for specifying coordination and composition of components [8, 10]. Due to the wide variety of events ranging from lower level physical signals to higher-level abstract events, CPS applications and users may be interested in certain conditions of interest in the physical world, according to which certain predefined operations are executed by the CPS. Detection of these conditions of interest (events) will lead to the desired predefined operations. As a result, any CPS task can be represented as an "Event-Action" relation [Tan09]. Some of the challenges involved in the representation events in dynamic real-time CPS are [NSF08]:

A. Abstractions for Sensors and Event Representations

Sensor data requires processing to generate information which can then be used for event identification and representation. Abstraction of sensor instances and event instances are required for representing sensors and events respectively. However, this is a challenging task that requires a framework that can deal with this problem in its entirety. Sensors can be represented as a resource with a unique identifier that allows them to be located through the Internet. In addition, it is important to develop the notion of: (1) Sensors classes which represent collections of sensors instances with particular properties, e.g. temperature sensors monitor and alarm class. This class could consist of several instances. To allow for mobility, this class would have both location and time as two amongst other properties; and (2) Event classes which represent collections of event instances with particular properties, e.g. intrusion event detection class which could consist of several event instances. Event classes too would have location and time (or at least position in a sequence in time) as two amongst other properties.

There will be relationships between these classes, which will allow for representation of generalization/specialization, composition and associations. As mentioned earlier, interoperability is an important challenge to be considered for the seamless integration of different high level applications. Successful implementation of this allows us to meet the following challenges: (1) Management of raw sensor data that is kept, maintained and exported by disparate sources; (2) Interpreting events associated with particular sensor configurations and outputs; (3) Transforming system level knowledge from distinct sensors into higher-level management applications; and (4) Upgrade of existing sensors with new advanced sensors using standardised interfaces by using the same abstract level representation.

B. Compositions of Sensors and Events to Address Complex Requirements

Depending upon specific application requirements, composition of event data from multiple sensors may be required. This is a challenging task that requires a dedicated framework on how information from multiple sensors is composed and correlated for meeting the QoS requirements of the specific application scenario.

A decomposition technique is needed for decomposing complex functionality into lower level resources which can then be met by specific sensors or events. This decomposition requires the specification of items in the aggregation and their dynamic sequence of execution or arrangement. The dynamics in the case of services can be modelled by using workflows specified in a language such as BPEL and in the case of resources by using Mashups which allow easier configuration of these workflows.

The composition of events remains a challenging issue with a focus on sequencing them to produce a composite event.

C. Semantics for Compositions of Sensors and Events

Semantics need to be provided for automatic sensor discovery, selection and composition. Semantics here is the study of the meaning of Things (resources that represent sensors) and events. It represents the definitions of the meaning of elements, as opposed to the rules for encoding or representation. Semantics describe the relationship between the syntactical elements and the model of computation. It is used to define what entities mean with respect to their roles in a system. This includes capabilities, or features that are available within a system.

Two approaches can be used to represent semantics. They are: (1) ontologies and (2) lightweight semantic annotations.

Ontologies are formal, explicit specifications of a shared semantic conceptualization that are machine understandable, and abstract models of consensual knowledge can be used. Using ontology, it is possible to define concepts through uniquely identifying their specifications and their dynamic and static properties. Concepts, their details and their interconnections are defined as an ontology specification. Ontology compositions are typically formed from many interconnected ontology artefacts that are constructed in an iteratively layered and hierarchical manner. It is necessary to use a graphical representation of ontologies at a higher level of abstraction to make it easier for the domain experts to capture the semantic richness of the defined ontology and understand and critique each model.

Ontologies can be used to define the following system properties: (1) Information and Communication, refers to the basic ability to gather and exchange information between the parties involved; (2) Integratability, relates to the ability of sensors and devices from different sources to mesh relatively seamlessly and the ability to integrate these sensors to build the final solution in a straightforward way; (3) Coordination—focuses on scheduling and ordering tasks performed by these parties; and (4) Awareness and Cooperation—refer to the implicit knowledge of the operation process that is being performed and the state of the system [Dillon09].

For representing the knowledge in a given domain ontologies and for adding semantics to individual resources annotation may suffice. A special challenge here is developing ontologies for events. Lightweight semantic RDF Metadata Annotations are an attractive alternative for providing semantics for CPS systems. The Resource Description Framework (RDF) provides an enhanced representation over XML including: (1) The triples (Resources, Property, Value) or (Subject, Predicate, Object), and (2) Defining relationships such as the concept of class and subclass.

RDF is extensible, which means that descriptions can be enriched with additional descriptive information. RDF is metadata that can be inserted into XML code or device or vice versa.

We discussed some of the features of RDF in Chap. 3. We briefly summarize or repeat them here in the context of providing semantics for CPS Systems. An example of an Extensible representation of a sensor instance is given in Fig. 8.5 and associated URL Hierarchy is given in Fig. 8.6.

Another important aspect here would be the use of RDF profiles (see Fig. 8.7 for Sample RDF Profile).

Semantics for CPS systems must be able to represent: Timeliness requirements; Resources descriptions (e.g. hardware or software applications); Quality of service; Schedule of tasks; and other functional issues that must be addressed. Thus, one can distinguish four main semantic components namely: Time—provides a detailed definition of time; Resources—provides a wide range of primitives for resource description including physical resources such as device, CPU or communication devices; As well as resource service such as application or services description; QoS—At this stage we have provided a profile for illustration of QoS concepts for

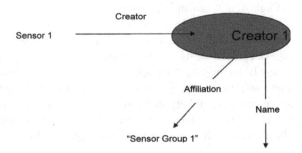

Fig. 8.5 Extensible RDF representation of a sensor instance

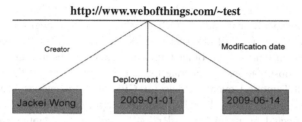

Fig. 8.6 URL hierarchy

Fig. 8.7 Sample RDF profile

Title	Definition
Identifier	An unambiguous reference to the resource within a given context
Description	Purpose of resource and what it does eg. measures xx quantity
Coverage	The extent or scope of the content of the resource
Creator	An entity primarily responsible for creating & deploying the resource
Format	The physical or digital manifestation of the resource
Date	A date of an event in the lifecycle of the resource
Type of resource	The nature or genre of the resource
Relation	A reference to a related resource
Access rights	Information about rights to modify & access the resource

Resource Instances description; and Causality—The description of action execution and resource service instance.

D. Event Models for CPS

Approaches have been proposed in the literature that model events in CPS. They classify events as temporal or spatial [Tan09]. They further define different dimensions such as (a) punctual or interval, (b) single or stream, (c) action or observation, (d) point or field, and (e) causal, discrete, or continuous [Talcott08, Tan09].

In a CPS, the events can be further categorised as follows [Tan09]: (1) Physical-events: Physical event models the occurrence of the end-user interest in the physical world and can be any change in attribute, temporal or spatial status of one or more physical objects or physical phenomena. These events are captured through physical observation, which is a snapshot of attribute, temporal, or spatial status of the target physical event; (2) Cyber-Physical events: The physical event captured using sensors collect the sensor event instances from other sensor motes as input observations and generate cyber-physical event instances based on the cyber physical event conditions; and (3) Cyber-events: The top level CPS control unit serves as the highest level of observer in CPS event model. It may combine cyber-physical event instances from other CPS components (sensors) and other control units as input observations to generate the cyber event. Some of these approaches utilise Spatial-Temporal event models for CPS in 2-dimensions [Tan09] and in another uses 3-dimensions [Tan10]. Another approach provides semantics to the events detected by using first order logic, such as an adaptive discrete event calculus [Yue10].

8.3.4.3 CPS for Emergency Monitoring and the Cloud

When we use CPS for emergency monitoring we note that there is:

- Less need for resources during normal operation
- A very large increase in Resources during emergency situations

  This also accompanied during the emergency situation by:

- Large increase in Data
- Large increase in needed Computational Resources

  This is necessary to:

- Identify type of problem being encountered
- Determine appropriate response to emergency identified

Hence, if the sizing of the capacity of computational resources was to meet the required resources during the emergency situation, the resources sit idle most of the time except during emergencies. There is, therefore, clearly a need for elasticity in use of computing resources. As elasticity is a key feature of cloud computing, the cloud combined with CPS is an effective approach to emergency monitoring.

In order to use Cloud for CPS for emergency monitoring, there is a need to have mechanisms for delaying all other tasks except those related to the emergency. Thus there is a need to build models of the real world and have these available for real time reasoning when the emergency strikes. This essentially requires the realization of:

"A Cloud of Things"

We have previously proposed the idea of a community of energy prosumers that negotiate with the utility for the supply to the utility and use of utility provided energy. Here again there is a necessity for elasticity and sharing of information across different prosumers. Here again the cloud of things has an important role to play [Dillon11a]. This can form a basis for the design of the proposed emergency monitoring Telemedicine system.

8.4 Conclusion

In this chapter, we first discussed the research and development underlying the Intelligent TCM Telemedicine System. This included the architecture, the ontology semantics, automated system generation and ontology evolution.

Next we examined the future directions for the work on the Intelligent TCM Telemedicine System including a Collaborative Multi Agent Recommender System, an Integrative Allopathic TCM Telemedicine System, Use of Cloud Computing and Cyber Physical System for the Intelligent TCM Telemedicine System.

In order to realise the full benefits of Cyber-Physical Systems, we need to have a framework that integrates various devices across the physical and digital domain on a real-time basis.

In addition, some functions in CPS require elasticity in availability of resources and here the cloud of things has an important role to play.

Among the various challenges, semantics handling and processing is an important one to be solved as it is the overarching element that provides context to the CPS events and operations.

To realize such a framework, we could utilize the Web-of-Things based framework in conjunction with the Cloud of Things that shows how all the various elements in CPS—Cloud Ecosystem interact.

References

[Armbrust09] Armbrust, M., Fox, A., Griffith, R., Joseph, A., Katz, R., Konwinski, A., Lee, G., Patterson, D., Rabkin, A., Stoica, I.: Above the clouds: a Berkeley view of cloud computing. EECS Department, University of California, Berkeley, Techical Report UCB/EECS-2009-28 (2009)

[Dillon09] Dillon, T.S., Talevski, A., Potdar, V., Chang, E.J.: Web of things as a framework for ubiquitous intelligence and computing. In: Zhang, D., Portmann, M., Tan, A.-H., Indulska, J. (eds.) Ubiquitous Intelligence and Computing, p. 213. Springer, Hiedelberg (2009)

[Dillon10] Dillon, T.S., Chen, W., Chang, E.J.: Cloud computing: issues and challenges. In: Keynote Paper, IEEE AINA 2010, Perth, Australia (2010)

[Dillon11a] Dillon, T.S., Potdar, V., Singh, J., Talevski, A.: Cyber-physical systems providing quality of service (QoS) in a heterogeneous systems-of-systems environment. In: Keynote, IEEE DEST 2011, Korea (2011)

[Dillon11b] Dillon, T.S., Zhuge, H., Wu, C., Singh, J., Chang, E.J.: Web-of-things framework for cyber–physical systems. Concurrency Comput Practice Experience 23(9), 905–923 (2011)

[Dillon12] Dillon, T.S., Jaipal, S., Hussain, O., Chang, E.J.: Semantics of cyber physical systems. In: Keynote IFIP Intelligent Information Systems, Guilin, China (2012)

[Lee08] Lee, E.: Cyber physical systems: design challenges. In: IEEE Object Oriented Real-Time Distributed Computing, pp. 363–369 (2008)

[Lee09] Lee, E.: Computing needs time. Commun. ACM 52(5), 70–79 (2009)

[Mell09]   Mell P., Grance T.: Draft NIST (National Institute of Standards and Technology) working definition of cloud computing—v15, 21 Aug 2009

[NSF08]   National Science Foundation.: Cyber-physical systems summit report, Missouri, USA. http://precise.seas.upenn.edu/events/iccps11/_doc/CPS_Summit_Report.pdf (2008). 24–25 April 2008

[Singh12]   Singh, J., Dillon, T.S., Hussain, O., Chang, E.J.: Event handling for distributed real-time cyber-physical systems. In: Keynote Paper, IEEE ISORC Conference 2012, China (2012)

[Talcott08]   Talcott C.: Cyber-physical systems and events. In: Wirsing, M., Banâtre, J.-P., Hölzl, M., Rauschmayer, A. (eds.) Soft-Ware Intensive Systems, LNCS, vol. 5380, pp. 101–115. Springer, Heidelberg (2008)

[Tan09]   Tan, Y., Vuran, M.C., Goddard, S.: Spatio-temporal event model for cyber-physical systems. In: 29th IEEE International Conference on Distributed Computing Systems Workshops, pp. 44–50 (2009)

[Tan10]   Tan, Y., Vuran, M.C., Goddard, S., Yu, Y., Song, M., Ren, S.: A concept lattice-based event model for cyber-physical systems. In: Presented at the Proceedings of the 1st ACM/IEEE International Conference on Cyber-Physical Systems, Stockholm, Sweden (2010)

[Yue10]   Yue, K., Wang, L., Ren, S., Mao, X., Li, X.: An adaptive discrete event model for cyber-physical system. In: Analytic Virtual Integration of Cyber-Physical Systems Workshop, pp. 9–15. USA (2010)

Printed in the United States
By Bookmasters